COLLINS GEM
ANTIQUE
MARKS
a mine of information

COLLINS GEM
B...
D0523615

COLLINS GEM
a mine of information

COLLINS GEM
CRICKET
a mine of information

COLLINS GEM
DIETING
FAT
a mine of information

COLLINS GEM
DOGS
a mine of information

COLLINS GEM
FIRST AID
a mine of information

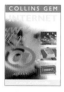

COLLINS GEM
INTERNET
Connect
a mine of information

COLLINS GEM
PREDICTING
a mine of information

COLLINS GEM
Ready
REFERENCE
a mine of information

COLLINS GEM
SHARKS
a mine of information

COLLINS GEM
WHALES
& DOLPHINS
a mine of information

COLLINS GEM
WHISKY
a mine of information

COLLINS GEM
WORD
PROCESSING
a mine of information

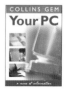

COLLINS GEM
Your PC
a mine of information

COLLINS GEM

SAS FITNESS

Barry Davies

HarperCollins*Publishers*

Barry Davies is an ex-member of the SAS, and the author of *Collins Gem SAS Self-Defence* **and** *Collins Gem Hillwalker's Survival Guide*.

HarperCollinsPublishers
Westerhill Road, Bishopbriggs, Glasgow G64 2QT

www.collins-gem.com

First published 2000

Reprint 10 9 8 7 6 5 4 3 2 1 0

ISBN 0 00 472483 6

Printed in Italy by Amadeus S.p.A.

Contents

INTRODUCTION

I served with the SAS for 18 years, of which I am justly proud. During that time I took a keen interest in hillwalking and survival, subjects I continue to practice and write about. Likewise, when I'm not writing, I shoulder my rucksack and taks to the nearby mountains around my home in Spain. When back in Great Britain, I often visit the Brecon Beacons and surrounding Welsh mountains to walk the same routes which I covered when I attempted SAS Selection – though, it must be admitted, at a more sedate pace.

> Losing weight, getting in shape and improving your lifestyle can only be done through self-motivation and will-power.

At the age of 54 and weighing some 16 stone 7lbs (104 kg) I decided to participate in my own fitness programme to achieve a better weight and standard of fitness. My progress is accurately recorded throughout this book and stands as testimony to its viability.

There is an old saying that 'life is what we make it'. That is to say, every individual can motivate themselves to achieve whatever they want. In many areas of our lives this, of course, is debatable, but when it comes to our physical health our fate really is in our own hands.

Recently, there has been a strong shift in adopting 'Boot Camp' military fitness programmes as an aid to exercise and slimming. As with most innovative ideas this started in the USA, but the concept has already caught on in the UK. Without doubt the British Special Air Service (SAS) are the fittest military unit in the world. True, there may be specialist individuals in the USA or Russia who could compete and maybe win, but as a whole, the SAS come out tops. This is not just my opinion it is also that of most other special forces units around the world. So how do they achieve this status? The answer is not pumping iron or working out in the gym for hours; it is a process called SAS Selection. Each volunteer who wishes to join must pass this course in order to be 'selected'.

As far as possible this book describes a set of programmes based on the principles of diet and weight reduction and the fitness requirements of SAS Selection. The programmes have been adjusted from their strict military structure, thus allowing anyone from 16 to 60 to participate according to their individual capabilities. For those who simply want to lose weight the book will show them how, and for those who want to achieve a phenomenal degree of fitness there is a full schedule based around the SAS selection process.

The procedures start with techniques to evaluate your present physical condition, then lay out a simple but enjoyable routine starting with short strolls and eventually leading to marathon-type walks across beautiful countryside. Just like SAS Selection, which takes six months to accomplish, your routine will be a gradual process but one that will achieve long-term results. If you feel the need to regain fitness or to discover the benefits exercise brings, then this is the place to start. Your reward will be a longer life, more stamina, a feeling of wellbeing and a healthy body.

WHAT IS SAS SELECTION?

Any soldier who wishes to join the Special Air Service (SAS) must first pass an extremely tough process called 'Selection'. A series of endurance tests ensures that only the best candidates make it through to further training. To begin with, any soldier applying for Selection needs to have had at least three years service with a parent unit, so that at least the basics of military discipline and procedures are understood. Many people imagine that only soldiers can apply to be part of the SAS, however, the Selection is open to all men in all branches of the armed forces, as long as they have served for three years.

Every SAS candidate will have to earn his place by proving his abilities. In this way no-one is actually picked or chosen by anyone else – it is merely a process of survival of the fittest. This practice ensures that successful SAS candidates tend to be highly motivated, highly focused individuals who are still able to work as part of a team. Once Selection has been passed, the candidate must then give up any rank previously held in his parent regiment and will once more become a trooper.

The Selection process itself takes place, for the main part, in the Brecon Beacons in South Wales. The Beacons are not particularly high, but the constant weather changes mean that they can be dangerous. More than one soldier has met his death through hypothermia. A prospective candidate needs to put himself through some

SAS selection requires that a soldier, who is already fit, pushes himself to the limit

sort of training schedule to get fit a long time before he gets to Hereford. The best way of building endurance is to go on increasingly long walks with a medium-sized rucksack. However, a good knowledge of map reading is also essential as the candidate will be required to navigate his own routes across the test sections.

The first obstacle encountered by the candidate is 'Test Week', which comes at the end of the first phase of SAS Selection. It is a week designed to test individual stamina and fitness and its gruelling nature often means that several candidates drop out every day. From my own experience, one of the best ways to make it through this week, apart from being fit, is to eat as much food as possible, especially breakfast. The finale of the week is a killer of an exercise known as the 'endurance march'. For this, the remaining candidates are expected to cover 25 miles (40km) in 20 hours carrying a rifle and a 55-lb (25-kilo) bergen, and, of course, the route is anything but flat.

The candidates start off in the early morning and will need to maintain a good, steady pace by walking uphill and running downhill. As the calorie burn during the march is high (estimated to be about 20,000), breaks for food need to be taken approximately every 3 hours for about 20 minutes each. Even then, the candidate is advised only to have a cup of tea and a light high-calorie snack as any heavier food will cause him to vomit when he starts off again. Boiled sweets can be sucked while on the move as these help to combat cold and fatigue; this is why they were originally included in military ration packs.

Summer Selection means that the candidate will be at risk of severe dehydration, while Winter Selection carries the threat of hypothermia. The soldier is expected to be aware of these dangers and to adequately safeguard against them. But whatever the time of year, he will still need to carry adequate protection against any sudden changes in weather. Thick fog, bad weather and darkness will all limit visibility, so a torch is a necessary item to be carried in the bergen. Another vital piece of equipment is the compass: the ability to work from a compass is invaluable when visibility makes normal navigation methods impossible. For those who can afford it, a Global Positioning System (GPS) may also be of use.

AUTHOR'S NOTE

When I joined SAS Selection I had been working out with a bergen for several months and considered myself fit. When I arrived at Hereford it was plain to see that many candidates had not bothered to exercise and as a result most were dismissed in the first few days. Not all of the overweight candidates failed as some, who I would call borderline cases, seemed to have the determination to keep going. One such candidate passed selection and remained with the SAS for 15 years, during which time he always looked fat and overweight. Yet this did not affect his fitness or make him slow during exercise activities. Looking overweight doesn't necessarily mean you're unfit.

Once the candidate reaches the end of the course within the allotted time, he will find army trucks waiting to take him back to base. The worst of the physical tests may be over, but there will still be much more training to come over the next few months before he will be able to call himself an SAS soldier.

AUTHOR'S NOTE

Don't worry, no-one is going to make you do SAS Selection, but we are going to incorporate many of its principles into our own fitness programme. These principles involve weight loss, fitness and endurance, all achieved through healthy eating, drinking and aerobic exercise. Whereas the SAS start off with professional soldiers, many readers of this book will need to find their own fitness level first.

SAS Fitness has four main levels. First, it concentrates on those people who are very overweight and are unable to exercise properly; those that consider themselves to be in this category will need to start with the Weight-loss Programme (page 57). The other three levels are based on simple fitness exercise programmes. The first concentrates on general health and fitness, while the other two are designed around the Special Forces Briefing Course and SAS Selection. Although these are modified for civilian use the routes are extremely gruelling. It is up to the individual to decide at which point they will enter a particular fitness programme, but I highly recommend that everyone undergo the health and fitness test prior to any strenuous exercise.

Before I became a writer I was extremely fit, running at least 20 miles a week and walking most weekends. However, along with the opportunity to change lifestyles, came the endless hours sitting in front of a computer (around 12 hours a day). Now some six years down the line and despite sticking to a rigid diet my weight has shot up, simply due to lack of exercise.

So during the three months it takes to write this book I will apply the same motivation and persistence to exercise as I do to my writing. (Before and after photographs along with a periodic weight check will be my affidavit to such.)

WEIGHTS AND MEASURES

The Imperial form is given first with the metric following in brackets. For example, weight is given in stones, pounds and ounces, with kilos and grams in brackets.

WARNING

The aim of this book is to help create a diet and fitness plan appropriate to an individual's current health and fitness levels. Everyone can aim for the same standards, with age, time and motivation being the only differences. This book is tailored to those of normal eating habits and does not cater for people on a restricted or specialized diet. It is not suitable for vegetarians or vegans. The diets and exercises described are for use in circumstances where safety or health are not put at risk. The author and the publishers will not accept any responsibility or legal liability for any health and fitness recommendations or diets used in this book. Individuals with heart and cardiovascular conditions, diabetes hypoglycaemia, kidney disease, stroke, gout, the very elderly, growing children, adolescents, pregnant women or anyone under medical care for any other condition must follow the dietary (including daily calorific intake) recommendations given to them or approved by their doctor, dietician, nutritionist or other qualified health professional.

A FIT AND HEALTHY BODY

DEFINING OUR AIM

It is sad to say that less than 30 per cent of the European population exercise on a regular basis; in the USA the figure is even lower. In itself this would not be so bad, but when you add a poor diet, the body becomes unfit and unhealthy. This is somewhat surprising given the benefits of a fit and healthy body. Improved cardiovascular fitness helps fight against heart disease, and weight loss improves energy levels as well as providing a feeling of wellbeing and a longer life expectancy.

How is this done? To start with you must ask yourself: 'What do I want to achieve?' Do you want to be slimmer? If so, by how much? Do you want to be fitter, and for what reason, e.g. to simply gain more energy or to run a marathon? Then ask yourself: 'What must I do to achieve that aim?' You must all answer these questions honestly.

The next requirement is to set yourself a realistic target, and a time span over which you can sensibly accomplish that target. In doing this consider how long it took you to gain weight or become unfit. Even with the best will in the world it's going to take a long time to reach your desired goal. Think about your age; we are all getting older and thus slowing down. Do you have the motivation? There can be no progress without a commitment to a long-term diet and exercise routine; many start off at a cracking pace but give up after a few days. There must be a determination to diet and exercise, in the same way as you commit yourself to go to work each day. Make time for your exercise programme and build it into your daily routine. This is particularly important during the first four weeks.

Defining Your Aim

Where you are now, and where you want to be in the future.

GETTING STARTED

Some basic knowledge of how the human body works is helpful if we are to get fit. We need to understand the benefits of proper nutrition and just how food affects the whole body. In particular it is crucial to know how the blood takes oxygen and nutrients via the heart to our muscles. These cause the muscles to develop healthily and to be able to stretch and contract properly, which, of course, enables us to move. In order for our body to be at its most efficient and vitalized, these processes must also be able to work at their optimum capacity.

However, it must also be understood that there are some differences in the physiological make-up of men and women, which must be detailed before we start.

Whether or not we like it, men and women are physically different.

DIFFERENCES BETWEEN THE SEXES

This book is aimed at both men and women and as such, the diet and exercise programmes are meant for both sexes. But there are differences which need to be taken into account when planning fitness goals.

BODY MASS

As a rule, most men have a greater body mass than women. For example, an average 18-year-old male will have a height of about 5 feet 8 inches (1.72 m) and will weigh around 10½ stone (66.15 kg). An average 18-year-old woman, on the other hand, will have a height of about 5 feet 5 inches and a weight of around 9 stone (57 kg). This difference will affect the amount of muscular strength between men and women.

MUSCLES AND BONES

In general, men have approximately 50 per cent more muscle mass than women as well as a greater bone mass. This means that although women are not as strong they do have greater flexibility.

FAT

The female body accumulates a greater amount of body fat than the male body. It is usually distributed in the buttocks, arms and thighs, whereas in men it tends to be on the back, chest and stomach.

HEART SIZE AND RATE

The heart of the average man is 25 per cent larger than that of the average woman and so is able to pump out more blood with every beat. This also means that men have a lower resting heart rate (five to eight beats a minute slower) than women.

LUNG CAPACITY

As with the heart, the lung capacity in men is about 25–30 per cent greater than that in women. This enables men to take in more oxygen when exercising.

THE HUMAN BODY

Our size and shape are mainly determined by our
skeleton, which is genetically inherited and sustained
by normal growth. While there is little we can do
about our skeletal frame, fat and muscle can be
altered because they respond to exercise. The
composition of the average human body is as follows,
though the percentages vary with age and gender:

- bone and minerals: 6–8%
- muscle and other lean tissue: 10–20%
- body fat: 15–25%
- water: 55–60%

THE SKELETON

Our skeleton is what provides the framework for the
rest of our body, both supporting and protecting
various parts of it. The size and shape of our skeleton
is genetically inherited but it can be influenced by
nutrition and disease. It contains a total of 206 bones,
half of which are concentrated in the intricate struc-
tures of the hands and feet. Various types of joints
connect one bone to another, making the body flexible
and able to perform a wide range of movements. Male
and female skeletons are similar but with a few slight
differences: the bones of the male are heavier and
thicker; while women have a shallower and wider
pelvis As already mentioned, the skeleton cannot be

altered (unless through disease, injury or surgery), but we can affect fat and muscle through diet and exercise.

MUSCLE

There are about 650 muscles in the body and they make up over 20–25 per cent of the total body weight, even in a newborn baby. They are generally attached to the skeleton by tendons. When the brain sends a signal along the nerves for a muscle to contract or relax, it does so, and the effect on its tendon and the attached bone causes that part of the body to move. However, it takes a whole group of muscles to move a part of the body not just one on its own. In a 'pull-push' process, one group of muscles will be relaxing while others are contracting in order to produce a movement. Exercise develops muscles and muscle groups either for stamina or for strength, depending on what kind of exercise is employed and therefore dictates our outer body shape.

BODY FAT

Body fat stores unused energy and is essential to a healthy body, but if it becomes excessive it can be unsightly and unhealthy. Women naturally carry more body fat than men, but both increase their body fat percentage with age. As a rough guide see table below.

BODY WATER

Water is the largest single component of the human body; the blood itself is 80 per cent water. The body has no way of storing water and so it constantly needs to be replaced by drinking fluids. This is why water is so important to health, and without it death will occur in about three days. Normal water loss occurs through the natural processes of respiration, urination and perspiration. Ideally, fluid intake should be equal to fluid loss; when we perspire or urinate we should drink in order to replace that loss on a regular basis.

AVERAGE PERCENTAGE OF BODY FAT

Age	17–20	21–27	28–39	40+
Male	20%	23%	26%	28%
Female	28%	30%	32%	34%

THE HEART

Of all the muscles in the body, the heart is the most important, for without it we would die. While we are alive, it works ceaselessly, pumping blood around the body; oxygen and nutrients are delivered to vital organs, bones and muscle, and waste products are carried away. The heart muscle is extremely efficient. It has four chambers: two of these deal with pumping de-oxygenated blood to the lungs for re-oxygenation;

while the other two receive the blood back from the lungs and pump it around the body. During activity or exercise, the heart needs to work harder to enable it to pump out more blood to the muscles. If these muscles do not receive the oxygen they require, they soon tire and build up waste products, such as lactic acid. Therefore, for improved fitness, the heart rate needs to be raised to 80 per cent of its maximum capability.

Like the rest of the body, the heart is vulnerable to injury and disease and the effects of these are potentially life-threatening. Heart, or cardiovascular disease can come in many forms and may be either mild or serious. Some forms are congenital but most are brought on by an unhealthy lifestyle and occur later on in life. A heart attack can be caused by diseased coronary arteries, cardiomyopathy, hypertension and valvular heart disease. Such conditions may be avoided by sensible diet and exercise. The twentieth century has seen many advances in the area of heart medicine, whether it be new drugs, pacemakers or surgical procedures. Many sufferers of heart disease have had their symptoms relieved or even eliminated altogether. However, the best cure is still prevention and the only way to do that is to keep fit.

The two main factors affecting the heart are diet and exercise. A poor diet over a long period causes a substance called atheroma to build up in the arteries. Eventually this wax-like substance will block the arteries and so interrupt the blood supply to that part

Keeping the heart fit can prolong life.

of the body. A blockage in the coronary arteries can cause chest cramps (angina) or even a heart attack.

As with any muscle the heart will respond and improve with exercise. A normal pulse rate is around 65–70 beats per minute. The resting pulse, taken when we first wake up, is normally a little lower. This resting pulse rate falls the fitter we become. In real terms this means the heart rate of an unfit person doing exercise will be around 120 beats per minute. In a fit person doing the same exercise it will be greatly reduced to around 85–90 beats per minute. In the course of a minute's activity the hearts of both the fit and unfit person will pump the same volume of blood, the difference being that the fit person's heart will need less beats to do it.

The unfit heart will simply beat faster to compensate for the exercise while the fit heart meets the demand by increasing the stroke volume – thus the fit heart does a lot less work. Getting fit also improves the blood flow around the body by lessening the resistance in the vessels and therefore lowering the blood pressure. A combination of high blood pressure and poor diet is the main cause of heart attacks.

THE RESPIRATORY SYSTEM

The respiratory system takes in oxygen from the air outside and supplies it to the blood. It is also responsible for the expulsion of waste gases such as carbon monoxide, which are a by-product of the respiratory process. Air is taken in through the nose and down to the lungs via the windpipe, or trachea. At the top of the trachea is located the voicebox, or larynx. Further down in the chest, the trachea branches into two tubes, called bronchi which lead into the left and right lungs. Within the lungs, the bronchi divide into smaller and smaller tubes called bronchioles. These all carry the air to tiny little chambers at the end of the bronchioles, called alveoli. It is in these chambers that the oxygen in the air is able to pass through the thin membranes of the walls and into the blood capillaries beyond. Here the oxygen molecules attach themselves

LEARNING TO BREATHE

If you have not exercised for a long time or are very overweight, you will have trouble breathing. Your lungs will need to expand again, which takes time and if you begin too quickly, you will suffer laboured breathing and chest pain. Control your breathing as follows:

• exhale fully, then inhale slowly to the count of 10;

• exhale to the same count;

• repeat this three times – it has an amazing effect. Once the burning pain has receded, carry on with the exercise but at a much reduced level of effort. If you still have chest pain remains, cease the activity and consult your doctor.

Fresh air feeds the blood that in turn feeds the muscle and brain. Work out in an area where the air is clean and vary the exercises so that the lungs operate at a variety of speeds. Once you have achieved a standard of breathing where you feel no undue pain or stress in the chest cavity, try to improve slightly by pushing yourself in short but vigorous exercise. The amount and quality of air we breathe has a direct effect on our health, as with the water we consume, purity and volume make for a healthy body.

to blood cells which then become re-oxygenated. In the same way, waste gases are able to cross from the blood and into the alveoli to be eventually expelled on the next outbreath. The lungs are able to inhale and exhale air due to the contraction and expansion of the thoracic cavity. This contraction and expansion is due for the most part to the workings of a large, thin sheet of muscle located just below the ribcage – the diaphragm, as well as the intercostal and abdominal muscles. The ribs themselves act to support and protect the thoracic cavity.

A CHANGE IN LIFESTYLE

There are other factors we must take into consideration when assessing our fitness which are not always readily apparent but are just as important. The major factor is our lifestyle. Work is the dominant part of almost everyone's lifestyle, with other periods such as sleep and leisure time falling into step. All of which make up our daily routine.

Changes to our lifestyles, our routines, can be difficult and often stressful, for example, a change of job. It is hard to uproot yourself and to head off in a new direction, and getting fit will certainly involve a great deal of alteration to your daily habits. However, concentrating on the benefits of being fit should provide you with the necessary motivation and determination to break your bad habits, and make getting fit and staying fit a central part of your way of life.

My own lifestyle has changed dramatically from soldier to that of writer

BAD HABITS

We all have some bad habits, such as excessive eating, drinking, smoking, or even, in some cases, drug abuse and dependency. No matter how you argue the case for alcohol or soft drugs, neither one of these promote a healthy body or satisfactory lifestyle. What we must recognize in ourselves is that the habit is there. If, like many people, you suffer from two or more habits then you have real problems. For example, if you drink and smoke excessively, the odds are you will die well before your time. The odd drink doesn't do much harm, but a build-up of alcohol in the system over years will cause irreversible damage to the liver, eventually leading to death. Excess alcohol also has a deleterious effect on the heart, kidneys, brain and other organs. There is no doubt about it that alcohol in large amounts is a poison to the system. Another toxic habit is smoking. The tar contained in cigarettes is drawn into the lungs and will eventually cause many major health problems. Heart disease, lung cancer, throat and mouth cancer, and thrombosis are all associated with smoking and all have a high death rate. Neither do you need to be a smoker to end up with the same disorders: recent research has shown that those people who constantly breathe in other people's smoke are also at risk.

If you feel that you could have a problem, do something about it. Plan to make a fresh start but do it slowly and tackle one problem at a time, whether it is your diet, smoking, drinking, stress or lack of exercise, and set yourself a simple goal to start with.

Bad habits can be hard to break but the benefits will make it worth it in the end.

THE BENEFITS OF FITNESS

Health and fitness help promote a long active life and, providing no major accident befalls you, if you resolve to make diet and exercise a long-term option then there is no reason why you should not achieve that aim. Fitness must become a part of your life, and the younger you start the better your body reacts.

Fitness not only controls your weight, but there is good evidence that you will be less prone to many life-threatening diseases, such as heart disease. Getting fit helps you to enjoy life a lot more; you feel better, have more energy and look a whole lot better too. The good thing about exercise is that you start to feel the benefits from day one. After four weeks you will find you have more energy and you will sleep better. Three months down the line and you will have improved your personal appearance, you will feel good and should have a lot fewer health problems. A year later, providing you are still keeping to your programme, your whole life will have changed and you will feel a different person.

MOTIVATION

Motivation is the process through which people provoke, endure and control what happens in their lives. In this case we are provoked to become fitter. For many of us this means having to endure a strict regime of diet and exercise while controlling the rest of our lives. One thing I promise you, no matter at what point in life you start your fitness programme, if you endure, you will reap the benefits. First you must understand why you want to be fit. For example:

- Do you consider yourself obese?
- Are you in poor health or do you have shortage of breath?
- Are you afraid that your partner is losing interest?
- Do you wish to feel attractive to others?
- Do you have the desire to run a marathon?

Study other people of the same age that you admire. What qualities do they have that you do not? Whatever it is, in the end it comes down to confidence and motivation and if they can do it, so can you. So how do you become motivated? In this case simply make yourself a promise: 'I will get fit.' True, that's the easy bit. Next you need the confidence to endure. Determination will help you on track – remember why you started this fitness programme in the first place.

DETERMINATION

For most of us getting fit is a long-term project, and your determination will require a boost from time to time. You may feel that all this training is getting you nowhere; why should you bother to continue? To this I can offer only one answer: get the first month over with, then your daily training will become second nature and before long you will start to enjoy it.

COPING WITH STRESS

Stress is an emotional and physical response to situations and events which we find unpleasant, worrying, annoying, frightening and so on; from traffic snarl ups to the death of a loved one, from a visit to the dentist to losing a job. However, it is an essential and natural part of life.

Constant stress over time can damage your health.

In many instances our body's reaction to it can be beneficial. Muscles become tense, increasing their flexibility and the breathing rate increases, so supplying more oxygen to the muscles. Sugars are discharged into the bloodstream to provide energy, and the heart rate increases to supply more blood to the muscles. Beads of sweat will break out from the skin, in readiness to cool the body as it overheats from strained exertion. If the stress is temporary, these symptoms will soon subside. However, if you remain in a 'wound-up' state over a long period, the biochemical state of your body will change and become unbalanced. It is thought that constant stress is the cause or at least a contributing factor in a range of health problems, such as temporary mental illness, certains cancers and heart disease. Fitness is one of the best ways of combating its effects.

AGE

No matter how strong your determination, motivation and confidence, the body ages and there is a point at which stage the ageing process will simply deny any further progress. As we get older we lose muscle weight, flexibility and the bones become brittle. When this will occur will differ in everyone, but it is often related to an individual's lifestyle. For some it will come early, while for others it may be in their seventies or eighties. There is little we can do about our age, but there is a lot we can do about showing it. To act young is to be young. Age brings many changes to our body but to some degree exercise and a healthy diet can counter the worst of these. Many men and women in their seventies and eighties still run marathons.

AUTHOR'S NOTE

During the 18 years that I served with the SAS I learnt many skills, most of which were totally irrelevant to civilian life unless I was going to use lock-picking and become a thief. However, during my service I was encouraged to return to night school where I studied and passed enough exams to get me into university. But more than any skill of academic achievement life in the SAS taught me two important things: you can be the equal of anyone, as all people share the same fears, doubts and hopes; and that though failure and despair have many depths, they can be overcome through motivation and determination.

MY OWN CHANGES IN LIFESTYLE

1–15: Born into a farming family. Fed on basic but good food, which consisted mainly of dairy products. Secondary Modern education. Three brothers and two sisters to play with. Simple life, little stress.

15–17: First job as an apprentice butcher boy working long hours, six days a week. Life was new, but uneventful. Diet change which included a higher meat intake. Little or no exercise. Discovered girls and sex.

17–22: Joined the Welsh Guards. Exciting, active days, travel and lots of group exercise. Diet change to three solid meals per day, and start of regular alcohol intake. First signs of stress as I was sent abroad and separated from my family. First fired a gun in conflict at the age of 20. Learning to become confident.

22–40: Volunteered for the SAS. Passing the Selection course was the most gruelling thing I have ever done. I was encouraged to remain fit for the rest of my service. Diet of little or no consequence. Travelled the world. Involved in several battles, got shot in the leg. Short periods of temporary combat stress. Confidence and motivation levels at maximum.

40–49: Set up a survival business, got divorced, made and lost a fortune. Fitness up and down like a yo-yo. Rich diet due to business trips and meetings. Quick weight gains and losses, health problems starting to show. Confidence took a hell of a hammering, but motivation stayed intact.

49–55: Became a full-time writer. I loved it so much I sat and wrote almost every day – result, no exercise. Too much rich food and alcohol. Health problems associated with being overweight. Confidence level returned to normal but motivation has slipped due to the 'good life'.

UNDERSTANDING WEIGHT CONTROL

In order to achieve fitness we must also understand the effect of food in relation to our weight. This is equally as important as exercise, because if an individual is vastly overweight they cannot exercise sufficiently enough to make any significant difference to their fitness. Eating appropriately is critical for the proper growth and functioning of our bodies. Understanding why we eat and the properties of what we eat is, in the long term, more important than exercise, but the best option is a balanced combination of both.

DIET AND EXERCISE

By reducing your calorific intake (eating less) and increasing calorie burn by expending more energy (exercising), you should realistically expect a weight loss in the region of one or two pounds a week. It is not wise to try and lose weight by dieting alone, however, because the body will begin to think it is being starved and will compensate in other ways. It does this by slowing down its metabolic rate and as a result tends to conserve fat so that weight is lost very slowly. It is also a myth that diets should be a form of starvation. The body needs a minimum of around 1500 calories a day to function properly, though certain people may require more or less due to special circumstances. Also, it is nutritionally sensible that the calories should be spread out over all the major food groups.

Crash diets involving food regimes that work on a smaller calorie intake a day are best avoided as these tend not to produce lasting weight loss. They simply deplete body water and lean muscle tissue rather than body fat. The best diets take time and are usually combined with some form of exercise so that muscle tissue is maintained while fat is reduced. Aerobic exercise is the best type of exercise for reducing fat as the oxygen used is also necessary for the metabolization of fat into energy. Exercises considered to be aerobic are: jogging; swimming; walking; dancing; aerobics; cycling; stair-climbing; cross-country skiing; rowing; and skipping. Whichever diet-and-exercise method you intend to use, it should be carried out in a safe and sensible fashion.

WHAT IS FOOD?

In order that we can live, the body must have air, water and food. As a guide, without air we will begin to die within four minutes, without water within four days and without food forty days. Air and breathing have already been covered in the previous chapter, and so now we will look at how food and water affect the body. The food that fuels the body falls into four main groups.

- Fruit and vegetables
- Cereals and breads
- Dairy products
- Meats

Eating a varied, well-balanced diet is as important as exercise.

EATING HABITS AND CRAVINGS

We eat when our bodies crave food either through hunger or because there is a chemical deficiency in our energy balance. We also eat for the pleasure of it, for the taste or socially, or we eat because we are feeling stressed. In the first instance, once our body is used to eating at regular intervals, such as breakfast, lunch and dinner, signals are sent to the brain close to those times demanding replenishment, and we interpret these signals as a craving. If we go without food for a long period of time, the signals become more intense until the craving is satisfied. It is known that a fall in blood sugar levels triggers the signal to eat, although a deficiency in one particular chemical, such as salt, will also cause a demand for replenishment. Failure to obey the warning may result in symptoms such as dizziness and weakness.

On average Westerners eat about a tonne of food each year, and usually it is a constant intake of high-energy and fatty food – and therein lies the problem. Eating a lot of food will not make you fat overnight; it takes time, years in many cases, for the fat to build. Equally, eating very little will not make you thin in a matter of days and your body weight will not fall dramatically. That is why when people start a diet their weight varies very little and they may become disheartened.

The secret to maintaining a stable body weight is to eat uniformly, matching your energy loss to your energy intake.

GUIDELINES FOR HEALTHY EATING

You should try to eat a wide variety of different foods from each main food group (see page 37), with lots of fruit and vegetables but smaller amounts of meats and other fatty foods. A wider variety of foods satisfies the appetite quicker and reduces the need for bulk. This variety will help provide the body with a sufficient amount of fats, proteins, carbohydrates, vitamins, minerals and water. While all are beneficial to health, the fat content of food is the most significant. The value of the food we consume is defined by its calorific value. Foods differ in the calorific energy they provide depending on the amount of fats, protein and so on that they contain.

> Once the principles of good nutrition are understood, maintaining a healthy, balanced diet becomes easy.

If the guidelines are kept to and food is selected sensibly, it will provide the body with all the nutrients it requires to stay healthy and without gaining weight. Ideally, we should eat three meals a day, perhaps with a healthy snack, such as fruit, in between. If such a regime is followed, most adults would not need any vitamin or mineral supplements.

WHAT WE EAT

The range and general quality of food has improved dramatically over the past 30 years, but this improvement has also increased the amount of appetizing, high-energy foods available and the desire to consume more. This can be clearly seen in the growth of supermarkets and the huge variety of food products they sell. In the 1950s our mothers would go to the grocers and choose from a comparatively limited selection of food, today we simply push our trolley down the aisle past a seemingly never-ending display of mouth-watering products. Today, it is not just a matter of buying something to eat but increasingly it's a case of 'oh that looks nice lets try it'. To maintain a well-balanced diet there are a few guidelines to follow when shopping for food. (A comprehensive list of calorific values is given at the end of this book.)

- Buy fresh food whenever possible, frozen if not.
- Select foods which can be grilled or boiled (avoid fried food).
- Avoid chocolate, ice cream and anything with a high sugar or salt content.
- Skip the aisle with the high-calorie soft drinks and spirits.
- Limit the amount of pre-cut chips.
- Avoid high-calorie 'pick-at' foods, such as peanuts.
- Make a shopping list and stick to it.
- Increase the amount of vegetables you eat and decrease the meats.
- Buy more fruit.
- Buy spring water and plenty of it.

Always try to buy fresh food, especially fruit and vegetables – apart from anything else they taste so much better.

FOOD USAGE

The bulk of what we eat falls into proteins, fats and carbohydrates, which make up over half of our daily energy requirement. The energy requirement is measured in calories. For a woman the average intake should be 2000 calories a day, for a man 2500. The ideal combination is 15 per cent protein, 35 per cent fat and 50 per cent carbohydrates. This roughly equates to:

- Breakfast: cereal with banana and skimmed milk, cup of tea/coffee with one sugar.

- Lunch: tuna sandwich, can of coke, piece of fruit.
- Dinner: lean steak, vegetables, cheese and biscuits.
- Drink: two measures of alcohol.

The importance of eating a well-balanced diet both in terms of differing foods and total quantity must be fully understood, especially when it comes to fat.

FATS

Fats are made up of carbon and hydrogen molecules. They differ in composition, but when considering health they fall into two main categories: saturated and unsaturated. In either case the more fat a food contains the higher the calorific value. The difference is that saturated fat will increase the cholesterol level in the blood, whereas unsaturated fats will help reduce it. The densest saturation takes place when a carbon atom is encompassed by the utmost number of hydrogen atoms possible. In general animal fats are highly saturated, while vegetable oil contains unsaturated fats. For example, butter is around 80 per cent fat of which 50–60 per cent is saturated, while a margarine high in polyunsaturates is 100 per cent fat of which only 25 per cent is saturated. It should be noted that we need to consume all fats, albeit in the correct amount, if we wish to maintain a healthy body.

EXCESSIVE FAT INTAKE

If we, as many of us do, eat until we have had our fill and ignore the content of the food we consume, then we will certainly include an excessive amount of fat in our diet. Excess fat makes your heart and vital organs work a lot harder. It blocks the arteries and restricts the blood flow, is unsightly and extremely heavy.

Body fat is accumulated over a number of years. There is a slow build up of layer upon layer until we

CHOLESTEROL

Cholesterol is a waxy substance that is vital to the walls of all body cells. Most cholesterol is manufactured by the body, mostly in the liver, with less than 15 per cent coming from our dietary intake. The more fat we eat, the more the liver is encouraged to produce cholesterol. Cholesterol has two forms: higher density lipoprotein (HDL) – 'good cholesterol'; and lower density lipoprotein (LDL) – 'bad cholesterol'. The difference being the amount of fat-laden protein attached. These are distributed around the body via the bloodstream and the related amounts of HDL and LDL are a good indicator of likely heart disease. It has been found that an increased amount of HDL has a beneficial effect on the body. To some degree this can be achieved by reducing the amount of saturated fats we consume in our diet. Additionally, HDL can be increased through exercise, though you will need to walk a total of at least 25 miles a week to produce a higher HDL level.

PROTEIN

Proteins form the structure of our bodies and without them we would dissolve into one big heap of goo. All our cells are protein based; they are essential for growth, cell repair and tissue replacement. Proteins are constructed from amino acids, so to make new proteins we need to eat foods that contain amino acids, such as fish, meat and eggs.

cannot ignore the problem. Even at this stage few people do anything about it other than to buy clothes in larger sizes. An increase in the amount of fat slows the body's functions, making the problem self-perpetuating as physical exercise becomes difficult, unappealing and even dangerous. Carrying surplus fat around also has a marked influence on breathing, which becomes ragged, short and rasping, preventing the body's metabolization of fat-burning oxygen.

CALORIE INTAKE

We eat food to sustain our bodily processes, which account for a little over two-thirds of what we consume, the remainder being used to fuel external activity, such as walking, working and exercise. If we do not eat enough while exercising extensively, we will burn off body fat – our body fuel reserves. If we eat too much and do not exercise then our fat reserves will get larger. Make sure that your daily calorie intake

CARBOHYDRATE

Carbohydrates contain atoms of carbon, hydrogen and oxygen in different configurations. These produce sugars and starches, the elements necessary for producing energy for movement in the body. When a carbohydrate is digested it breaks down into simple sugars, such as glucose, which can then be used by the body as fuel to provide energy for all the metabolic processes. Glucose does not just go straight into the blood; some of it goes to the liver where it is converted to glycogen and stored for future energy needs. Once these stores are depleted, the body will draw upon its fat and protein reserves to provide it with the fuel it needs. Carbohydrates also contain an amount of dietary fibre, but this is mostly removed during the body's processing of the food. Examples of foods high in carbohydrates are potatoes, wholemeal bread, pasta, rice and fruit.

is matched to your needs; you will need more food if you intend to go hillwalking than if you are sitting at a desk all day. The secret of maintaining a sensible weight is all down to balancing energy needs. The exact amount of food, and therefore calories, required to maintain an even balance will depend on our age and lifestyle. The older we become, the less energy is required to maintain body muscle. As our lifestyle changes, due to work practices and social activities, so will the amount of calories required to maintain that balance.

CALORIE BURN

A calorie is one-thousandth part of the heat needed to heat one litre of water by one degree centigrade. It is the energy value by which foods are measured when consumed. For fitness terms a calorie is the measured amount of energy that is released as heat when food is metabolized by the body. The amount of calories in various foods and drinks vary, but as a rough guide:

- Fat contains nine calories per gram.
- Alcohol seven calories per gram.
- Carbohydrates and protein four calories per gram.

The amount of energy an individual burns during a single day will depend on their activity and to some degree their exercising body weight. Most of us follow a daily routine which comprises of work, rest and play. For example, we all sleep for roughly 8 hours during which time the calorie burn is around 65 cph (calories per hour). As our work practices differ so will our calorie burn. For example, an office worker's will differ from that, say, of a farm worker. Most of us also spend a couple of hours travelling either to and from work, to the shops or to some leisure activity. The rest of our time is taken up with relaxation and personal activity. Our personal activity time is where we can make a major difference to our daily calorie burn. For example, a sluggish teacher who spends his activity time 'surfing the net' in the evening will have a total calorie burn of around 2760 calories per day, while a waitress who enjoys dancing will average over 4000 calories per day.

Typical Daily Calorie Burns

Sleeping:
65 cph x 8 hours = 520 calories

Travel time:
80 cph x 2 hours = 160 calories

Desk work, driving
100 cph x 8 hours = 800 calories

Hospital worker, school teacher:
200 cph x 8 hours = 1600 calories

Construction worker, waitress, farm worker:
250 cph x 8 hours = 2000 calories

ACTIVITY TIME

Work, travel and sleep make up the usual daily routine of most people. Activity time normally associated with the period after work and on the weekends is when we can make the largest contribution to our daily calorie burn. If we are involved in a non-physical hobby, such as the Internet, night school or watching television, we will add little to our daily calorie burn total. If, on the other hand, we go 'clubbing' several times a week, belong to a gym or play football on the weekends, our overall calorie burn will be dramatically increased. Raising the calorie burn during some of our routine activities can also be attained by short periods of greater activity. A good example is walking all or part of the way to work, or walking around the shops at lunchtime.

Sample activities and their calorie burn

Watching television, Internet	80 cph
Walking, dancing	250 cph
Jogging, tennis, cycling	300 cph
Running, football	400 cph
Bergen hillwalking, squash	500 cph

(A more extensive list is given at the end of the book.)

During any form of aerobic exercise, fat is only one source of energy used by the body: it will also use carbohydrates from any food consumed. This means that it can take a great deal of exercise to burn up a significant amount of calories. For example, it takes about a mile of walking at a normal pace to use up 100 calories. If you consider that there are 3500 calories in one pound of fat, this means it would take about 35 miles of running or walking to burn them off

FLUID INTAKE

Fluid intake is vital because all body functions use water, added to which water accounts for almost 60 per cent of our body composition. It should, however, be noted that fat cells hold the least amount of water, which means the fatter we are the less water our bodies contain and therefore excessive water loss will make little difference to body weight loss. Additionally, if we have a low water content then our body minerals will not dissolve properly throughout our circulation.

Thirst and hunger control our intake while the kidneys direct the bulk of body fluid output, thus our body's water supply is kept in balance. If we become

Drink plenty of water – two to three litres a day is recommended.

overweight or continue to consume too much of the wrong food and drink then we suffer an imbalance. There is a tendency with most people to forget the importance of fluid intake and the benefits associated with drinking fresh water. In general we eat less of those foods with a high water content, such as fruit and vegetables, cooked rice or pasta, in favour of foods with a low water content, such as meat and sugars. Additionally, we tend to drink more tea, coffee, soft drinks and alcohol than we do fresh water, and so most people live with a water imbalance.

AUTHOR'S NOTE

The extreme climatic conditions endured during my SAS days have left their legacy of severe arthritis in both my elbows and forearms, something I have endured since I was 30 years old. Over the past six months having replaced my tea drinking with water, the arthritic pain has all but disappeared. Whether this is down to my increased water intake I cannot say, but my gut feeling tells me it is.

FRESH CLEAN WATER

Drinking fresh water is just about the best thing you can drink to control the body's fluid balance. It will seem strange to begin with, but try replacing your daily cups of tea with water. At first you will find yourself drinking double the amount, which is good, and you will gain no weight. After the first few weeks your system will start to show the benefits, with a clearer complexion and a reduction in the amount of body pain encountered while exercising.

Depending on its source, water will differ in taste. Natural spring water is best and a large variety is available in all supermarkets. However, my advice is to do a little research at your local library and find out where the nearest natural spring is, then drive there and fill as many containers as possible. Consuming around three litres a day will result in a diminished craving for food and alcohol. It will aid sweating during exercise, making the skin healthier and the muscles supple.

DRINKING ALCOHOL

In addition to food and water most people consume varying amounts of alcohol. Due to alcohol's high calorific value, it has a significant effect on diet and fitness. As already mentioned, fat contains nine calories per gram, carbohydrates and protein contain four calories per gram but alcohol contains seven calories per gram.

Small amounts of alcohol drunk occasionally do little or no harm, and there are those who consider that small quantities are actually beneficial. By and large, drinking falls into two categories: drinking for pleasure or reward, or drinking to fulfil a dependency.

Drinking occasionally and in moderate amounts will have no effect on your physical fitness, but those with alcohol dependency put themselves at risk because exercising with a high blood alcohol content can cause death. The amount of alcohol in the bloodstream also affects our behaviour; the more we drink the less control we have. However, although alcohol makes us talkative, uninhibited and stimulated, it is in fact a depressant. Spirits are absorbed quicker than beer, and fizzy mixers only help to speed up the process. Eating will slow down the rate at which alcohol is absorbed into the bloodstream, and the more weight we carry the longer it will take for alcohol to have any effect. As a rough guide the blood alcohol level per 100 ml of blood will be as follows.

- 1 pint of beer or 2 shots of spirit = 30 mg
- 2 pints of beer or 5 shots of spirit = 60 mg
- 5 pints of beer or 12 shots of spirit = 100 mg
- A bottle of spirits drunk within 4 hours = 400 mg

Even at 60 mg judgement can be defective and we start to lose discrimination and common sense. At 100 mg balance, vision and muscle control are all affected. For those on a bottle a day, death is not far away.

The point at which people switch from being a social drinker to one dependent on alcohol is a very grey area. For the most part people have an inbuilt regulator, and soon realize by their increasing number of hangovers and lack of concentration that they are drinking too much. The problem is further compounded by building up a tolerance to alcohol which means that increased amounts are required to achieve the same effect. This is the first sign that we are on the road to life-threatening alcohol dependency. In this event you are faced with one option – stop drinking.

Excessive drinking is as damaging to your health as smoking.

REDUCED ALCOHOL INTAKE

The relationship between alcohol and fitness is a balance, but quite simply the less you drink the fitter you are. If you drink too much alcohol then you need to bring your drinking under control. If you drink to excess, you will need to abstain altogether. If you drink socially, as most of us do, but feel you can control your drinking, you should still try to restrict the amount of alcohol you consume. You need only come up with a few reasonable excuses.

- I'm driving.
- I'm on prescribed drugs.
- I have a liver problem.
- I can't drink at lunchtime it makes me sleepy.
- Turn up late at parties and go home early.
- Drink mixers only and pretend they contain alcohol.
- Drink only every other day.
- Drink a glass of water between every alcoholic drink.

GO DRY

In the context of this book the only real option is abstinence. If you are only a social drinker then this will not be a problem. For those with a heavier consumption, it will do them the power of good to stop. The weight you lose when not drinking is a major bonus in itself.

Most of us like a drink and in moderation it can be beneficial, or so I am led to believe. But often the problem is what we perceive as moderation. A serious taste for alcohol starts in our late teens; by our mid-twenties social activities demand that we can hold our own with the best of them. From our mid-thirties onwards most of us start drinking excessively. That is to say, we fall into the trap of drinking every day and it becomes a habit just like smoking. Ask yourself a few questions.

- Do you drink some form of alcohol most days?
- Do you wake up with a hangover at least once a week?
- Is your concentration at work and in the home falling off?

If the answer to any of these is 'yes' then you have a problem – how big a problem only you really know. If you can't stop it yourself, and you are the best judge of that, get help. See your doctor, or better still join Alcoholics Anonymous – these people offer advice and help that works.

WEIGHT-LOSS PROGRAMME

The Weight-loss Programme is mainly aimed at those people (including myself) who are so far overweight that strenuous exercise is both impracticable and dangerous. This doesn't mean we cannot exercise, it simply means we must first correctly adjust our body weight. The programme also is an excellent guide for those who simply wish to lose weight. For those very overweight I suggest that you repeat this programme until you have achieved your desired goal.

To start with, be honest with yourself and define what stage you are at now, then set yourself a target. This means determining your body weight and fitness levels as well as examining your daily routine, both at work and at home. It also means taking a good look at your diet and lifestyle, such as drinking and keeping late nights. Another consideration prior to embarking on a weight-loss and fitness programme is your age – will your body stand it?

Exercise is only one part of the equation when it comes to getting fit: nutrition is just as important if the body is to perform at its maximum potential. The following chapter aims to set out the basic principles of nutrition and give guidance for achieving weight control and strengthening physical performance.

EATING HEALTHILY

In the UK and USA there is a great deal of talk about eating healthily but few people lead by example. However, this is not true of all nations. For example, in the Mediterranean countries most people eat a well-balanced diet, and the beneficial results are clear to see. I do not say that such eating habits are a deliberate attempt to diet, more that circumstance and nature

Fresh fish and seafood should be part of everyone's diet.

have provided a range of staple foods that are very healthy as well as being native to the region. Most of the Mediterranean coastal area is one large garden, producing a wide range of fruit and vegetables, olive oil and fish. The abundance of free spring water in most towns and villages and the added bonus of clean, dry air also undoubtedly help.

LIFESTYLE EATING

The way we eat and what we eat is directly related to our social circumstances and lifestyle. Some people will eat only fish and chips or beans on toast because that is all they can afford, while others will eat the same merely from habit or because it is the easiest option. At the other end of the scale, being in the position to buy expensive business lunches or indulge in exotic foods is no guarantee that you are providing your body with a well-balanced diet. In addition to individual circumstances and lifestyle there is the added media pressure of what is good or bad for us, according to the latest research. 'Don't eat butter it's really bad for you.' 'Eggs will give you salmonella.' You may think it madness to ignore professional medical opinion but recently my mother recalled that as a young girl, between the wars, she had helped her granny make enormous breakfasts for the farmer husband and his workers. These included eggs, home-cured fat bacon, toast and lashings of home-made salty butter – and there was still lunch and the evening meal to go. It was a time when farming was still very

AUTHOR'S NOTE

Before moving to Spain I tried several diets but they did little. I simply stayed the same weight or became heavier. But four months in Spain and I have lost three stone – why? Diet, fresh air, water and exercise in that order.

The diet was not planned but just included local foods, mainly fresh fish, seafood and salads. Cooking was all done by grilling or with virgin olive oil; the latter was also mixed with a little vinegar to make the salad dressing. At least 90 per cent of the meals were cooked outdoors, barbecue style. Due to the heat most Spaniards spend a lot of their time sitting outdoors. The heat makes you sweat, and the need to slake your thirst is constant. There is local spring water freely available and a constant supply of fresh orange juice, either from the local trees or the supermarket. So I drank a great deal more of both than I used to. Also, keeping to the exercise programmes in this book encouraged me to walk the local mountain paths or go for a bike ride along the quiet roads, which became more of a pleasure than a chore.

Despite this sounding like a promotion for everyone to live in Spain, the point I am trying to make is that these factors really do promote a healthier lifestyle and a natural loss of body weight.

labour intensive and farm workers worked long hours. Butter, full-cream milk, home-made bread all saturated with salt and fats were the mainstay diet of most of my fore-family, many of whom lived into their late nineties. My mother is now 80 years old and she still dances, goes shopping on her bike, has an active brain and frequently travels abroad. The point she was trying to make is: it's not what we eat, it's is how well our body converts the food energy we supply it with. Life today is much easier than it was in 1925. Our day-to-day physical workload is less demanding and to compensate we must live on a diet free of fat and dairy products in order to keep our cholesterol in check.

Hamburgers, eggs and chips may look and taste good, but the meal shown here is more than 2000 calories.

OBESITY

Obesity poses a serious health risk. There is only one real answer to the problem and that is to lose weight. Other than surgery the only way to achieve this is to consume fewer calories and steadily increase the amount of aerobic exercise taken. If you do not have the will-power to do this then you may need to find a partner or join a diet organization. Even if you do join a group, you must still make time in your home life for regular exercise as this will help keep you on track when your group course has finished.

The advantages of reversing the effects of obesity are numerous – a slimmer more attractive figure, a fitter and more agile body and a better lifestyle overall. What must be kept in mind is the time span over which any weight loss should occur. Because someone who is obese is unable to participate in strenuous exercise the initial weight loss will be achieved through diet. This involves keeping strict control over calorie intake while maintaining the body's nutritional requirements. How much we need to lose and over what period of time can be discovered by simple mathematical equations – see the box opposite.

Another more simple way of assessing weight is to grab the skin at the side of your waist between your fingers and thumb without pulling. Measure the over-hang of skin and estimate the depth. If its more than a centimetre

Body Mass Index (BMI)

BMI is defined as your weight in kilos divided by your height in metres squared. The recommended BMI in women is set between 18–23, while in men it is 21–26.

For example, for a woman who is 5 feet 6 inches tall and weighs 12 stone 5 lbs the calculation would be:

77.85 kilos ÷ 2.72 m (1.65 × 1.65) = 28.62

(to convert lbs to kilos multiply by 0.45; to convert inches to metres multiply by 0.025)

The upper BMI limit in women is 23, which when subtracted from 28.62 leaves 5.62. This figure multiplied by the height squared, 2.72, equals 15.28, which is the number of kilos she is overweight.

The recommended weight loss per week is 2.25 lbs (1 kilo), therefore it will take some 15 weeks for her to achieve her goal.

thick you are carrying excess fat. To estimate the amount ignore the first 2.5 cm (1 inch) then multiply every centimetre over by 10 kg (22 lb). For example, if your skin pinch is 5 cm (2 inches) in total you will be roughly 25 kg (55 lb) overweight.

AUTHOR'S NOTE

When I joined SAS Selection I had been working out with a bergen for several months and considered myself fit. When I arrived at Hereford it was plain to see that many candidates had not bothered to exercise and as a result most were dismissed in the first few days. Not all of the overweight candidates failed as some, who I would call borderline cases, seemed to have the determination to keep going. One such candidate passed selection and remained with the SAS for 15 years, during which time he always looked fat and overweight. Yet this did not affect his fitness or make him slow during exercise activities. Looking overweight doesn't necessarily mean you're unfit.

WEIGHT-LOSS REGULATION

Weight-loss and physical-training programmes for overweight people can only work through regular exercise and reduced calorie consumption. The type of exercise we undertake affects the amount and nature of the weight loss. Both running and walking burn about 100 calories per mile. One pound of fat contains 3500 calories. Thus, burning one pound of fat through exercise alone requires a great deal of running or walking. On the other hand, weight lost through dieting alone includes the loss of useful muscle tissue. Those who participate in an exercise programme that emphasizes the development of strength and muscular endurance, however, can actually increase their muscle mass while losing body fat. These facts help explain why exercise and good dietary practices must be combined.

It is possible to determine how much excess weight we are carrying and adjust our calorific requirements to safely and successfully lose excess fat. We can also devise a sound individualized exercise plan which will develop useful muscle tissue while increasing fat loss. Generally, overweight people should strive to reduce their fat weight by 2.25 lbs (1 kilo) per week. However, it should be remembered that when we start to lose weight, either by diet or exercise or both, a large weight loss is not unusual. This may be due to water loss associated with the using up of the body's carbohydrate stores. Although these losses may be encouraging, little of this initial weight loss is due to the disappearance of fat. Weighing under similar circumstances and at the same time each day will accurately monitor progress. This helps avoid false measurements due to normal fluctuations in body weight during the day. As a person develops muscular endurance and strength, lean muscle mass generally increases. Because muscle weighs more per unit of volume than fat, caution is advised in assessing a person's weight loss progress. Just because a person is not losing weight rapidly does not necessarily mean they are not losing fat. In fact, a good fitness programme often results in gaining muscle mass while simultaneously losing fat weight. If there is reasonable doubt, the percentage of body fat should be determined and a revised fitness programme begun if need be.

One good idea is to keep a calorie control chart in your kitchen. As you prepare or eat food mark down the quantity and the calories. This will give you an understanding of the food value and help you regulate your diet. Fresh fruit need not be counted in this chart, but it should be considered as a perk. Likewise, the best way to monitor your progress is to get a calendar and fill in the weight each day. If you don't want anyone to know about your diet or see your progress keep it in a safe place.

Estimating Your Present Condition

For the purpose of this book it is argued that three overriding factors govern our lives: age, health and weight. If you are 22 years old, of average height, with no illness and weigh around 11 stone (if you are a man) or 10 stone (if you are a woman) then you have no problem. If on the other hand you are 55 years old, average height with a slight heart problem and weigh 16 stone, you need to think about weight loss before starting any serious exercise. The following is a rough guide as to what you can expect from your body through different ages.

Aged 18–25

This is when the body is at its peak of fitness. Most people in this age group find natural fitness through a healthy social life. Dancing, late nights and an active sex life make for a high calorie burn.

26–36

This is the time when most people get married. A supply of steady work is required to protect the family interests, such as paying the mortgage and seeing to the family's needs. Stress can become a health factor. The body's fitness is still maintained by the demands of home-building.

36–45

The risk of heart disease starts to increase. This is the time when the body's calorific needs start to decline and the weight goes on. Daily alcohol intake may increase. This is an important time to review one's lifestyle. Fitness now needs constant attention and work – social sports, such as football and squash will help.

46–60

Heart disease is the main killer, but if you take up steady exercise again, it is possible to improve your lifestyle. Long walks, gardening, and a careful diet will help maintain your fitness.

cont

---

60 plus

This is the stage where your previous lifestyle catches up with you. If you have abused your body then you will start to suffer now that you are older. If you have had a healthy life then there's no reason why you should not live to a ripe old age. Continue eating a healthy diet and take daily exercise.

PERSONAL ASSESSMENT

This is the moment of truth. If you have purchased this book and are serious about getting fit or losing weight then you must first assess your present condition. The best way to do this is to stand naked in front of the mirror and turn around slowly. Next, to confirm your worst fears, step onto the bathroom scales and weigh yourself. Then work out your excess fat using the BMI method on page 63 and compare the results with the Height to Weight Chart opposite. (Note: If you have a small frame then deduct 4½ lbs (2 kg) from the range, if you have a large frame, add 4½ lbs (2 kg) to the range.)

DO YOU WEIGH TOO MUCH?

If you are within the BMI range and your weight and height fit in with the chart, give or take a few pounds, then you don't really need to follow the Weight-loss Programme and can proceed straight to Programme

Weight to Height Chart

Men		**Women**	
Height	Av. Frame	Height	Av. Frame
5' 4"	9–9.3 st	4' 11"	7.4–8.2 st
(1.62 m)	(56.5–62 kg)	(1.52 m)	(46–51.5 kg)
5' 5"	9.2–10 st	5' 1"	7.5–8.4 st
(1.65 m)	(57.5–63 kg)	(1.55 m)	(47–52.5 kg)
5' 6"	9.4–10.4 st	5' 2"	7.8–8.6 st
(1.68 m)	(59–65 kg)	(1.57 m)	(48.5–54 kg)
5' 7"	9.8–11 st	5' 3"	8–8.9 st
(1.70 m)	(61–69 kg)	(1.60 m)	(50–55.5 kg)
5' 8"	10–11 st	5' 4"	8.2–9.2 st
(1.72 m)	(62.5–69 kg)	(1.62 m)	(51.5–57 kg)
5' 9"	10.3–11.3 st	5' 5"	8.4–9.4 st
(1.75 m)	(64.5–71 kg)	(1.65 m)	(52.5–59 kg)
5' 10"	10.3–11.3 st	5' 6"	8.7–9.4 st
(1.78 m)	(66.5–72 kg)	(1.68 m)	(54.5–61 kg)
5' 11"	10.6–11.5 st	5' 7"	9–10.4 st
(1.80 m)	(68–75 kg)	(1.70 m)	(56.5–65 kg)
6' 0"	10.9–12 st	5' 8"	9.3–10.7 st
(1.83 m)	(70–77.5 kg)	(1.72 m)	(58–67 kg)
6' 1"	11.2–12.4 st	5' 9"	9.6–11 st
(1.85 m)	(72–79.5 kg)	(1.75 m)	(60–69 kg)
6' 2"	11.5–12.7 st	5' 10"	9.9–11.2 st
(1.88 m)	(73.5–82 kg)	(1.78 m)	(62–70.5 kg)
6' 3"	12.1–13.4 st	5' 11"	10.1–11.5 st
(1.90 m)	(76–84 kg)	(1.80 m)	(63.5–78 kg)
6' 4"	12.5–13.8 st	6' 0"	10.4–11.8 st
(1.93 m)	(78–86.5) kg	(1.83 m)	(65–73.5 kg)

One (page 86). For those who are half a stone (3.1kg) overweight first get a checkup from your doctor to make sure you are fit enough to start exercising. Only then should you proceed to Programme One. If you are more than a stone overweight, any exercise will carry the risk of serious injury as the added weight will impose extra strain on joints, and increase the already overworked organs such as your heart and lungs. Sudden, enforced exercise on an overweight body can lead to a heart attack. Consult your doctor and carry out the Weight-loss Programme first.

WARNING

Do not conduct the following fitness test if you have recently suffered from any illness, have heart problems, are taking prescribed medication or have been drinking heavily within the past 24 hours. Check the following questions and seek qualified medical advice if the answer to any is 'yes':

Do you suffer from heart problems?

Do you have high blood pressure?

Do you suffer from chest pains?

Do you suffer from dizziness or regular headaches?

Do you have a medical condition that prevents exercise?

Are you on medication?

Are you 30 years or older and new to fitness?

Are you seriously overweight?

FITNESS TEST

Being of normal weight for your stature and height does not automatically mean you are fit, it simply means you are not carrying excess fat. Having established your weight you now need to determine your present standard of fitness. This is a simple process whereby you monitor your heartbeat both at rest and during a set activity.

Start your fitness test by checking your resting heart rate.

RESTING HEART RATE

Sit quietly in a chair and relax for a full five minutes. Then check your pulse rate by placing two fingers on the carotid artery in your neck or on the inner wrist. Count the total number of beats for 30 seconds then double the number – this is your resting heart rate. The average is around 75 beats to the minute. Slightly lower is excellent, but if your count is 85 or higher then you could have a problem.

STEP TEST

Find a step not less than 12 inches (30 cm) but not more than 16 inches (40cm) high. Start stepping up and down at a non-stop, steady rate for 5 minutes. Stop, sit in a resting position and take your pulse rate for 30 seconds, doubling the number to calculate for one minute. The average should be around 140 beats. Lower is good but any higher and you are unfit.

BLOOD PRESSURE

Go to your doctor or practice nurse and get your blood pressure tested. Don't worry about being a pest as most surgeries encourage people to have a checkup. A normal person in their mid-thirties will have a blood pressure of around 120 over 80, but the doctor will indicate any risk if different.

The photograph above is me at the start of this book, weighing 16 stone 7 lbs (105 kg). That's around 4 stone (25.5 kg) overweight for my height.

TYPES OF FITNESS

There are several types of fitness, including aerobic, anaerobic, isometric and isokinetic. The range of exercises involved in fitness varies from walking (aerobic) through to using weight machines in a health club (isokinetic). Although all are beneficial, the aim of this book is to concentrate primarily on aerobic fitness through simple exercises such as walking, running and hillwalking with a bergen (rucksack), following a similar structure to that of SAS Selection.

Likewise, this book is based on a long-term (six-month) exercise and diet routine. The platform for this programme is to build on progressive aerobic exercises to the point where you feel confident to tackle some serious fitness work. The range of aerobic exercises is fairly diverse, however, those chosen are simple, work extremely well and require the minimum of equipment. In addition to the walking, step-ups and sit-ups illustrated in the Weight-loss Programme we are going to add skipping, press-ups and jogging. All are designed to increase breathing and muscle activity.

AEROBIC AND ANAEROBIC EXERCISE

An aerobic exercise is one which is sustained steadily for a duration of time, typical examples of such exercise are walking, running and swimming. These activities steadily increase the intake of air through the lungs while breathing. Anaerobic exercise, on the other hand, involves short bursts of activity, for example, tennis and football. These activities mainly use the oxygen which is stored in the muscles. In this book, for the most part, we will concentrate on aerobic fitness, which is aimed at increasing the heart rate. This increased heart rate, if sustained for 45 minutes or more, helps prompt the heart to grow more muscle, therefore next time we exercise we should find it marginally easier. A continuation of this process is known as 'physical fitness'.

Aerobic exercise is best for burning fat.

Physical Fitness

Prolonged physical fitness increases the efficiency of the heart and lungs, which help to deliver oxygen and nutrients needed for muscular activity. Muscular strength is also improved, allowing muscle groups to be exerted for a longer period. The ability to move the joints or any group of joints with a greater degree of flexibility through a normal range of motions becomes easier while body fat is depleted.

Eight-week – Two Stone Weight-loss Routine

The following weight-loss programme consists of diet and light exercise. Its purpose is to reduce body weight to the point where strenuous physical exercise will cause no harm or undue strain on bone or muscles. The programme will work best if you incorporate it into your daily life. The foods listed below are only a guide, you may select different foods as long as they contain roughly the same calorie count and you include a wide variety to ensure you get all the necessary nutrients. Keeping a daily calorie intake and weight log are essential.

This eight-week weight-loss routine is designed to reduce your calorie intake while gently getting your heart and lungs pumping and your muscles working. The diet is not excessive, just choose any one of the seven choices or similar for each of your three daily meals. You may have the same meals twice in the same week if you so wish. The breakfasts and lunches are straightforward but follow the instructions for preparing the dinner menus in the chapter on diet. Again, providing the calorie count is similar, you may devise your own meals (a list of foods and their calorific values can be found at the end of this book).

The physical workout is not difficult and consists mainly of walking, step-ups and sit-ups. The programme can be completed in 30 minutes and should be carried out in the morning and early evening. Where possible they should be incorporated into your daily routine.

GROUND RULES

- Calorie count all your meals. Maximum 1500 calories per day for men, 1300 for women.
- No eating or snacks after 6pm in the evening (water consumption only).
- No alcohol for the first week and then mid-week only thereafter; maximum of five measures over the weekend. Avoid spirits if at all possible.
- Drink at least two litres of water per day.
- Eat at least two pieces of fruit a day.
- Prepare and cook fresh food whenever possible.
- Don't skip an exercise because of the weather.

Sample Breakfasts

One boiled or poached egg on one slice of toast
Bowl of cereal with fresh fruit and skimmed milk
Toast spread with either Marmite or honey
Bowl of fresh mixed fruit
Half tin of beans on toast
Half a honey-dew melon
Yoghurt

Sample Lunches

Vegetable sandwich: beetroot, cucumber, tomato,
    lettuce, cold potato
Home-made soup
Fresh fruit

Sample Dinners

Tuna or boiled egg salad
Cauliflower cheese with plain rice
Fitness Stew (see page 185)
Whole trout with salad
Liver casserole
Slice of tortilla (Spanish omelette) and salad
Sausages and mash

Soft Drinks

Drink as much **water** as you like (spring water is
best). Add a small amount of Ribena or similar to
add appeal if you find it bland.

Pure **orange juice** from the supermarket is fine but
freshly squeezed is nutritionally better. Half a glass
per day maximum.

One glass per day of **skimmed milk**, including what
you use on your cereal.

Alcohol

No alcohol for the first week then limit yourself to a small amount each evening. Avoid all spirits and drink low-alcohol long drinks such as beer and cider. They will quench your thirst and your compulsion. No lunchtime drinking allowed.

LIGHT EXERCISES

As well as the diet it is important to start exercising. This will not involve anything strenuous but will help start to develop muscle tone and get you ready for a regular fitness routine. You should complete two sessions, one in the morning and one in the evening. Always relax before you start and let any food to digest for at least an hour. The walks and steps required during the first four weeks are purely to get you moving. Any set of steps inside or outside your home will suffice. The walks should always start and end at your front door and have a purpose if possible, such as going to the shops or walking the dog. Keep the walks as flat as possible and if you must walk uphill, do so slowly.

WARNING

If, due to your weight, you are unable to carry out these two simple exercises then you should seek medical attention.

Walking

For most of us this natural exercise accounts for most of our daily calorie burn. For this reason those who walk or move around on their feet all day will generally be a lot fitter, such as a postman or nurse.

The average person carrying no load should be able to walk at a pace of around 3.5 miles per hour over flat ground. According to your abilities, start off by walking at a slow pace, increasing speed and stride as your body gets warmer. You do not have to make a special effort to maintain a walking routine, it can become part of your daily travelling, for example, walking to and from work, or walking to the shops instead of taking the car.

The premise of this whole book is based on walking and as the weeks go by you will be able to increase your duration and start to walk over the countryside and hilly terrain (see Programme Two, page 107). Building on this, you will eventually be able to walk some 12 miles (20 kilometres) over the mountains carrying a heavy rucksack.

Step-ups

Just like walking, most of us climb one or two sets of stairs during the day. This is an excellent form of aerobic exercise, but you should start off slow and build up carefully. Of all the aerobic exercises, steps are about the most beneficial while your body is over-weight. The number of steps you need to exercise on can vary from 1 to 100, although a set of 10 is just about perfect, just walk up and down normally. However, doing step-ups for exercise does not require a flight of stairs as one step between 10–12 inches (25–30 cm) high will suffice. This can be a bench, concrete block or door step. The exercise is easy: step-up one foot after the other, then step down and repeat. Whatever number you climb the initial pace should be set at 50 steps per minute, descents not included. For example, if you have 10 steps in your flight you will need to climb and descend them 6 times in a minute. Increase the number and speed of the steps you do in a session, as you feel able. Step-ups help strengthen the calf and thigh muscles.

Step-ups can be done by everyone including the overweight.

SIT-UPS

For those who wish to lose weight sit-ups are probably the best form of exercise because they improve the strength of the abdominal muscles. As with other exercises there are many varieties, but for the benefit of this book we will stick to two methods.

Lie down flat on the floor. Place your palms over your ears, with your elbows running parallel down your chest. Raise the head and shoulders together until the upper arm is resting on your chest (placing your hands behind your head increases the risk of damaging your neck and back muscles); relax and repeat the movement. Try to avoid getting into a 'rocking motion' as this reduces the efficiency of the exercise.

The author hard at work! To avoid possible strains while doing sit-ups, buy an abdominal exerciser.

A far easier way to benefit from sit-ups is to purchase a purpose-built abdominal exerciser. These are little more than a support for the neck and shoulders because the weight is lifted by your hands pulling on a rocker-type bar. With this apparatus the number of sit-ups can be greatly increased without putting undue strain on the neck and back. Although these abdominal exercises will not reduce your weight by any significant amount they will firm up the muscles, making you look slimmer and thus feel better.

First Month

Week 1 – exercise everyday

Morning:	Evening:
2 x 50 steps in 2 min.	Repeat morning exercise

Rest
1-mile walk

Week 2 – exercise 6 days, rest 1

Morning:	Evening:
3 x 60 steps in 3 min.	Repeat morning exercise

Rest
2-mile walk

Week 3 – exercise 6 days, rest 1

Morning:	Evening:
4 x 70 steps in 4 min.	Repeat morning exercise

Rest
3-mile walk

Week 4 – exercise 6 days, rest 1

Morning:	Evening:
5 x 80 steps in 5 min.	Repeat morning exercise

Rest
4-mile walk

Second Month

Week 1 – exercise 6 days, rest 1
Morning: Evening:
5 x 80 steps in 5 min.   Repeat morning exercise
Rest; 2 x 20 sit-ups;
Rest; 2 x 20 press-ups;
4-mile walk

Week 2 – exercise 6 days, rest 1
Morning: Evening:
5 x 80 steps in 5 min.   Rest
Rest; 3 x 20 sit-ups;
Rest; 3 x 20 press-ups;
4-mile walk

Week 3 – exercise 5 days, rest 2
Morning: Evening:
5 x 80 steps in 5 min.   5-mile walk
Rest; 4 x 20 sit-ups;
Rest; 4 x 20 press-ups;
5-mile walk

Week 4 – exercise 5 days, rest 2
Morning: Evening:
5 x 80 steps in 5 min.   Repeat morning exercise
Rest; 5 x 20 sit-ups;
Rest; 5 x 20 press-ups;
5-mile walk

By the end of the two-month programme you should be doing 4000 step-ups, 1000 sit-ups, 1000 press-ups and walking 50 miles per week. This equates to a calorie burn of around 7000 calories or 2 lbs of fat. If, in addition, you stick to the above diet for the two months you will lose at least two stone in weight. To reduce your weight further simply repeat week four of the second month.

Exercise Partners

For many of us, losing weight starts off as a very personal thing due mainly to our public declaration that we are unfit or overweight. While you may wish to exercise alone, you will achieve far better results if you choose to exercise with one or more partners. The advantages are enormous, none more so than the maintenance of motivation. When you feel like giving up, your partner should impel you into continuing, and vice versa. Additionally, a common bond will develop that makes the routine more of a social pleasure than an individual endeavour. Some of the rewards of having good partners are:

• Shared motivation
• Good reliance on routine
• Stricter weight control
• Reduced exercise boredom
• Reduction in stress levels

Listening to music

Listening to music or an instructional tape is a great way of taking your mind off the monotony of your morning jog or exercise routine. However, it does present several dangers. First off, running on a public highway while listening through a headset prevents you from hearing the traffic. Switch off and remove the headset wherever vehicles or moving machinery are present. Second, beware of the dangers of trying to stay in time with music or video exercises which have a fast beat.

Listening to music can inspire and get you through some of the monotony of exercising, but take care when near to traffic.

PROGRAMME ONE

GETTING FIT

If you have managed to comply with the Weight-loss Programme, or were one of those fortunate people who were the correct weight to begin with, it is now time to start getting fit. By completing the Weight-loss Programme, or at least by staying within 80 per cent of it, you will have accomplished several important things. You will have achieved the discipline of a regular routine and from here on in exercise will get easier and become more enjoyable. Providing you have stuck to the dietary requirements, you will have flushed your system with water and reduced your dependency on alcohol. Your breathing should be easier, making your muscles more active which in turn will add to your feel-good factor. But your main reward will be when you step on the scales. If adhered to correctly for the full twelve weeks, the programme will produce a body weight loss of 20–24 lbs (9–11 kg).

If you are new to exercise, or have just finished the Weight-loss Programme, set your exercise goal at around 50 per cent of what you would like to achieve for the first few months. As your heart rate and breathing improve increase your goal to 75 per cent. If you are still overweight then continue repeating the last week of weight-loss exercises until you reach your target weight, then move on to Programme One.

AUTHOR'S PROGRESS

I am now one month into writing this book and have kept to the strict diet and exercise programme detailed in the Weight-loss Programme. The feel-good factor hit me when I weighed myself and found that my weight had fallen from 16st 7 lbs (105 kg) to 15st 11lbs (100 kg) – a loss of 10 lbs (4.5 kg). I checked the scales for several days after and my weight fluctuated no more than a couple of pounds either way. As I looked in the mirror I promised myself that by next month I would crack the 14-stone barrier. The problem remaining is one of bodyweight: I am still too heavy to start strenuous exercise. I am repeating the Weight-loss Programme for another month with the addition of two sets of floor exercises, which are designed to increase muscle strength and improve flexibility. What pleases me about the Weight-loss Programme is the fact that I do not feel as if I have deprived myself of any food – I have simply taken control of what goes in my mouth.

MAINTAINING CALORIE INTAKE

Before we start our first exercise programme there are a few things to understand. These are fairly simple rules which will help guide and maintain your progress. In addition, you need to understand how to carry out each exercise properly and for the right duration. For those people who have completed the Weight-loss Programme, remember to stay within the height-to-weight guidelines (page 69). Moreover, calorie intake can rise to help balance the energy output as you increase your amount of physical exercise.

The Amount of Calories You Need

To find out the amount of calories required to maintain your ideal weight convert your ideal body weight to pounds and multiply by 15 – this will give you your daily calorie intake. This is based on a moderately active person; those who do less exercise or physical work will require less and vice versa. For example, a nurse of medium build weighing 9st 2 lbs will require 1920 calories per day (128 lbs x 15) to maintain her ideal weight.

GENERAL FITNESS RULES

The two most important rules are: first, to set aside time for exercise and so build it into your lifestyle; second, to maintain a regular routine you must avoid injury, the chances of which can be reduced by warm-up exercises (see opposite).

FREQUENCY OF TRAINING

It is the frequency of training which determines how fit you will become and how long you remain fit. The more exercise you do the fitter you will become until you reach your peak, or desired goal. This programme starts off by exercising every other day for periods of around one hour. After three weeks this is increased to five times a week with two rest days evenly spaced. There is also an increase in the duration of each session to around 90 minutes.

Once your fitness goal has been achieved you may wish to advance to a higher degree of fitness, or choose to switch to a more social form of exercise, such as squash. Frequency of training is best recorded in your weight and fitness log. This means you can keep a check on your progress and so help prevent you slipping back into old habits.

WARM-UP EXERCISES

The importance of warm-up exercises cannot be overemphasized and need only take a few minutes. Setting off cold will increase the risk of damage to joints and muscles. To begin your warm-up routine I suggest you do the following:

1 Start by deep breathing, fully exhale, then inhale slowly to a count of 10

2 Exhale to a count of 10

3 Repeat this three times

The purpose of this is to increase the amount of oxygen being delivered to the muscles, which in turn produce energy. Deep breathing will also help you relax and make your body go loose.

Most warm-up exercises have been around for many years and are common sense. Depending on how you feel, spend around 30 seconds to a minute on each exercise. Start off gently, working all your muscles through the full extent of their function, speed up slightly as your heart rate increases. The exercises below cover most of the basic muscle movements.

ARMS

1 Stand straight and circle your arms above your head like a windmill. Reverse every 15 swings.

2 With arms out at 90 degrees from the body, rotate the arms in a small circle. Reverse every 15 swings.

TRUNK

1 Stand straight with the left arm out at 90 degrees and the right arm folded across the neck. Turn the trunk while flinging the arms in a scythe-like motion from side to side. Reverse every 10 swings.

2 Stand straight, hands on hips and dip from side to side: 10 times each side.

3 Stand upright and stretch your arms into the air above your head. Bend your knees, bringing your arms down in front of you between your legs, and touch your toes. Return to the standing position. Repeat 5 times.

LEGS

1 Stand on one leg while raising the other knee and hugging it to your chest. Pull for about 5 seconds, let go and do the same with the other leg. Repeat 5 times with each leg.

2 Stand on one leg and grip the ankle of the other behind you, pulling it into your buttock. Pull for 5 seconds, then change legs. Repeat 5 times with each leg.

3 Find a wall or a tree and rest your palms flat against it. Open your legs to your normal stride, keeping your feet flat on the ground. Bend the inner knee so that the calf muscle of the trailing leg is lightly stretched. Hold for 10 seconds and switch legs. Repeat 3 times each leg.

4 Find a bench or wall around waist height and place

one of your legs on it. Stretch forwards from the waist touching your toes with your hand until you feel a slight strain. Hold for 10 seconds then change legs. Repeat 3 times each leg.

5 Lower yourself from the standing position to a squat then stand up. Keep your back straight all the while. Repeat 5 times.

6 With your feet slightly apart, bend your knees and stretch backwards with one leg, while bending the other knee. At the same time raise your elbows above your head, forcing them backwards slightly. Repeat 3 times with both legs.

SAS TIP

One of the best ways to start off a warm-up session is by running on the spot. If you choose to listen to music while warming-up make sure that the tempo is not too quick; the idea is to relax.

SKIPPING

Skipping is a low risk, aerobic exercise that can be done by almost anyone, no matter what their weight or lack of fitness. It can be made as hard or easy as it needs to be. Athletes and performers of all kinds, from boxers to ballerinas, use skipping as part of their work-outs. This is because it provides hard exercise but without the risk of serious injury. Unlike jogging or running, skipping is regarded as a low-impact exercise.

The other advantage is that it only requires a skipping rope and a flat surface – no fancy equipment or expensive gym membership. The best type of rope to buy is a professional leather rope, which are inexpensive, are of the right weight and long-lasting. Even those who are as yet unable to jog or go on long walks due to breathing difficulty will still be able to participate gently in this exercise.

Skipping is one of the best and safest of aerobic exercises.

Start off slowly and aim to jump just high enough to clear the rope as it swings under your feet. Try and keep a constant rhythm without faltering for at least a minute then have a little rest. Once you have your breath back, skip again for another minute. Persistence will help to build up the lung capacity and muscles, and you will soon be able to skip for longer and longer. Once you are really proficient, try taking the knees higher as well.

Skip with both feet together or by taking running steps. Beginners tend to find it easier to run lightly on the balls of their feet, but once you get faster, jumping with both feet together on the spot will most probably be the preferred option. The rope itself should be swung by rotating the forearm and the wrist only, and making sure that the rope just skims the ground. At first many people leave the rope too slack, which then bounces on the floor and becomes tangled with the feet. Make sure that your elbows are tucked firmly into your waist and that you stand straight, with your shoulders back and your head up.

Once you have reached the stage where you feel you have settled into a steady routine and speed, you should then attempt to do four sessions of between two and three minutes within an hour. This will not only greatly improve your lung capacity but it will also build up the muscles in your calves and lower legs – which will be a great benefit when you get on to the hillwalking.

PRESS-UPS

Press-ups could be called the mainstay of fitness – certainly as far as most armed services are concerned. Again, like all exercises, press-ups can be easy or hard but the important thing is to do them correctly.

1 Lay face down, arms bent in the frog position, palms flat on the ground directly under the shoulders, body flush to the floor, legs and feet together.

2 Raise your head, look forward and gently ease a rigid body off the floor using your arms. The position is correct when both the arms and body are straight.

3 Relax in a controlled attitude by bending your arms back to the frog position.

The single most common mistake that is made by beginners is allowing the stomach and hips to sag. Although this will have the effect of making the exercise easier, it also removes 90 per cent of the benefit which defeats the whole object and makes the exercise pointless. Press-ups can be varied in a number of ways. For example, the feet can be raised on a step or low chair, or the hands can be placed closer together under the upper chest, both of which require a lot more effort.

You can do press-ups almost anywhere, all you need is a space that is as long as your body. Also, for such a simple exercise that requires no equipment, they work a whole range of body muscles from the neck down to the toes. If you are fairly new to exercise, start with just 10 press-ups and repeat as you feel able. When you feel fit enough increase the number to four bouts of 25 spread over your training session.

SAS FITNESS DEFINITIONS

BEST EFFORT

Best effort means just that, giving it 100 per cent plus. Always make sure that you have warmed up properly before starting out on a best-effort run, and that you cool down after. As with all the exercise tasks, start off at a good but controllable pace, speed up and then push yourself to the limit for the final third.

HILL REPETITIONS

Find a steep slope, which is at least 200 metres long with an incline of around 30 degrees or more. It should take no more than a minute to sprint to the top. Sprint up the hill, then jog down to recover. Hill reps are designed to build your leg power and lung capacity. One hill rep is classified as 'sprint up, jog down'. Take short sharp steps and lean into the hill, relax as you jog down.

HOW TO RUN

It may sound silly but many people have forgotten or don't know how to run properly. The first thing to do is make sure your footwear is suited to the terrain you will be covering; blisters can be extremely painful (see Boots and Footwear, page 140).

Run with your body in an upright relaxed posture and let your arms adopt a natural swinging motion between your waist and chest. Run lightly making sure that your footstrike hits the ground with rhythmic timing. Shorten your step on the incline and extend it slightly on the decline. If your route takes you over uneven ground, be careful to avoid stepping on loose or protruding objects. Don't run too fast; you should be able to talk while running.

The terrain over which you run should also be considered. Remember we are not trying for Selection, so there is no need to take a dangerous route over rocky or marshy ground. Choose your route for its even pathways, its scenic beauty and its ease of access. If the route has very steep inclines then vary your pace accordingly.

JOGGING

Jogging is little more than fast walking and the secret of jogging is duration, not speed. Time on your feet is what's important. Start your jogging programme only after two weeks of walking, especially if you are new to fitness. Once you start jogging, concentrate on a pace that suits you. Jog with a heel first action, letting the toes claw into the pace and push off with the ball of your foot. Jog within your breathing capabilities, that is, run at a pace where you can hold a normal conversation.

MARCH

The SAS terminology for walking with a bergen over the hills. Try to maintain a steady pace, walking all the time. Don't be tempted to run down hill during your build-up training, it is the easiest way to injure yourself.

NORMAL RATE

Run at the same pace making sure you can maintain a steady rhythm to your breathing. This should be about 70–80 per cent of best-effort pace.

ORIENTEERING

Running at normal pace while following a set route around given points. It is is used to develop map and compass skills. Introduce this type of training into your programme at the earliest opportunity.

PACE

- Walking pace should average 18 minutes per mile.
- Jogging pace should be around 12–15 minutes per mile.
- Slow Running 10 minutes per mile.
- Normal Running 8 minutes per mile.
- Short fast run 5–6 minutes per mile.

POINTS ON RUNNING

Running is a simple aerobic exercise that raises your heart rate, increases oxygen intake and improves blood flow. It will tone muscle and reduce body fat. However, you must run to suit your body weight; the heavier you are the slower you should run. After a while, the more weight you lose the faster you can go. The reason for this is simply to avoid injury.

REPETITION TRAINING

Run over level ground at your best effort for 1 minute, then jog for one minute. Start by doing this 3 times, building up to 6 of each. Once you can run and jog comfortably for 1-minute intervals, increase the distance to 90 seconds and so on.

SAS TIP

During SAS Selection, I found that the best way to face a route was to split it into quarters. For the first quarter I would go slow, getting used to the bergen weight and letting my muscles warm up. For the second I would settle down, pick up a little speed and take a moment (still walking) to admire the view. By the third quarter I was focused on speed and timings, and put all my effort into completing the course on time. Sometimes during the last quarter there would be time to slow down towards the end so that when the DS decided to send you off on another route immediately you could comply.

Five-week Normal Fitness Programme

Week One

Monday–Friday
Morning:
3-mile walk;
skip for 3 min.;
2 x 20 press-ups;
2 x 30 sit-ups

Evening:
Repeat morning exercise

Saturday
Morning:
5-mile jog

Evening:
Rest

Sunday
Morning:
Rest

Evening:
Rest

AUTHOR'S PROGRESS

I am now into my second month, having repeated the Weight-loss Programme while I was writing this chapter. I have lost almost two stone since I started, but am still a little overweight. I now feel ready to participate in regular physical exercise. The sit-up machine has proved a great bonus as it has firmed up my stomach muscles giving me a much slimmer profile. My next goal is to complete the Five-week Programme, finishing with a 15-mile mountain walk.

Week Two/Three

Monday
Morning:
5-mile jog

Evening:
Swim 15 lengths

Tuesday
Morning:
5-mile jog

Evening:
Skip for 10 min.

Wednesday
Morning:
3-mile best effort

Evening:
Skip for 10 min.

Thursday
Morning:
5-mile jog, best effort

Evening:
Swim 15 lengths

Friday
Morning:
20 hill reps of
200 metres

Evening:
Skip for 10 min.

Saturday
Morning:
3-mile best effort

Evening:
Rest

Sunday
Morning:
Rest

Evening:
Rest

Week Four

Monday
Morning:
5-mile jog
(increase speed)

Evening:
Swim 15 lengths

Tuesday
Morning:
Skip for 10 min;
3 x 20 press-ups;
3 x 30 sit-ups

Evening:
Repeat morning exercise

Wednesday
Morning:
Rest

Evening:
Rest

Thursday
Morning:
5-mile jog, best effort

Evening:
Skip for 10 min.

Friday
Morning:
5-mile jog

Evening:
Swim 15 lengths

Saturday
Morning:
Rest

Evening:
Rest

Sunday
Morning:
Rest

Evening:
Rest

Week Five

Monday

Morning:
6-mile jog & walk
with rucksack
Time: 1 hour 45 min.

Evening:
Skip for 10 min.;
3 x 20 press-ups;
3 x 30 sit-ups

Tuesday

Morning:
Rest

Evening:
Rest

Wednesday

Morning:
8-mile jog & walk
with rucksack
Time: 2 hours 15 min.

Evening:
Rest

Thursday

Morning:
5-mile jog, best effort

Evening:
5-mile comfortable jog

Friday

Morning:
Rest

Evening:
Swim 15 lengths

Saturday

Morning:
10-mile jog & walk
with rucksack
Time: 3 hours 30 min.

Evening:
Rest

cont

Week Five (cont)

Sunday

Morning:
15-mile jog & walk
with rucksack
Time: 3 hours 30 min.

Evening:
Rest

ALTERNATIVE EXERCISES

The basis of this book is to get fit while walking and running. However, from time to time there may be reasons why neither can done. It is therefore a good idea to have some form of back-up exercise, such as swimming and cycling. The frequency and duration of these exercises will depend on how long you cannot walk or run. If your programme has been interrupted due to an injury, see your doctor to check if you are fit enough to swim or cycle. Always make sure that any injury is fully healed before continuing a rigorous fitness programme.

SWIMMING

Apart from running over the hills every SAS soldier entering the Regiment must pass a basic swimming test. In the beginning this test is normally swimming fully clothed in the local baths, but later the annual test is often done by swimming a mile in the sea. For those who cannot swim there is usually a crash course.

If you cannot swim, you are advised to go to your local swimming pool and enrol for a course. It is normally not expensive, and the students are put into groups according to age. The basics of swimming can be learnt in just a few lessons and improved at your leisure.

As with cycling there are several advantages of swimming. It is possible to swim while suffering from some form of injury as the water supports the body's weight. Swimming is also excellent for asthma sufferers as it does not provoke exercise-induced asthma.

Moreover, to get any real fitness benefit from swimming you need to swim relatively fast for at least half an hour at each session. While simply swimming up and down may feel good it will do little to improve your fitness. You should give yourself a time limit, for example, 30 minutes, and see how many laps of the pool you can achieve in that time.

Swimming is an excellent form of exercise, with the added advantage that it supports the body and so it can still be done by someone carrying a minor injury.

CYCLING

Cycling is not part of SAS Selection, but is an excellent alternative to running. Indeed, you can cycle when suffering from leg strains caused by running. The distance covered on a bike is roughly five times that of running, although both are achieved with the equivalent energy burn.

Choose where you cycle with care. Cycling in traffic is dangerous and unpleasant, while mountain biking is very prone to accidents. A hard-surface route fairly free of traffic is ideal. You must always wear a cycling helmet. If you intend to do long distances on a racing bike, padded shorts are essential, also a water-bottle.

As with running, it is time in the saddle that is important. If you are not used to cycling, take it easy to start with, and make sure the bike is adjusted to suit your body and pedal stride. Begin with short (five-mile) routes and build up the distance slowly. This will give the muscle groups around the upper thigh and buttock time to become active. Get used to anticipating the inclines and declines ahead of you and so adjust your gearing.

Cycling can be a sociable as well as effective exercise.

PROGRAMME TWO

Soldiers who wish to join the SAS must first spend a weekend at Hereford where they are briefed on the qualities required by the SAS. This briefing takes place some six months prior to the soldier actually attending Selection and gives them time to achieve the required fitness level. The following chapter is loosely based on the fitness schedule issued on the Special Forces Briefing Course (SFBC). Those who have completed Programme One of this book should now be ready to tackle some serious training.

Unlike the earlier programmes where the maximum effort was a fast jog, now you have to run. Run fast, run uphill, run downhill, run in the rain, snow and sun and run with a bergen. It sounds arduous and that's because it is. However, taking into account that we are not actually joining the SAS, we can modify the programme to make it much more enjoyable. We can do this by choosing our own routes and setting our own times and goals. But these goals must be met.

NEW TO HILLWALKING

In the normal course of events hillwalking is not dangerous, on the contrary in many ways it is far safer than the cities. It is purely the isolation factor that presents any great threat, but as long as a few simple rules are obeyed you should have no problem. If you opt for a pre-planned route, such as from a guide book, then any problems will be indicated and the appropriate action obvious. If you have chosen your own route, you should make sure you don't put yourself too far from safety. If possible:

- Never travel alone.
- Always tell someone sensible where you are going and your estimated time of return.
- Always have a contingency plan for bad weather.
- Carry a first-aid kit.
- Carry a mobile phone if you have one.
- Do not take unnecessary risks.
- Learn to read a map and use a compass.
- Dress and carry the appropriate clothing and equipment.

GOOD NAVIGATION

It is important to master both map reading and navigation skills if you intend to participate in cross-country exercises similar to that endured on SAS Selection. Not only will such skills reduce your chances of getting lost, they will also enable you to find the shortest way and the best terrain to get from one point to another.

Navigation can be done in two basic ways. The best known and the most traditional is to use a map and a compass. A more modern method is to use the technical advantages of the Global Positioning

A map is essential for hillwalking.

System. Although the latter may seem more appealing, bear in mind that it can be costly and if the batteries run down at an inopportune moment, you could be in trouble. Therefore, though both methods are covered here, more emphasis will be put on the proper use of a map and compass. This skill, whether you use GPS or not, is an important one and should be learnt by anyone taking part in any outdoor fitness pursuit.

ORDNANCE SURVEY MAPS

Without a good map it is easy to get lost in the countryside. For example, a right of way may become obscured by undergrowth and crops, but a map will be able to show you where it should be. Of all the maps available the best are Ordnance Survey (OS) maps, because these are often more detailed than those found in guide books and the like. Ordnance Survey maps come in different scales; most commonly 1:50,000. While these are good in their own right and show the public rights of way (marked in red), the

AUTHOR'S NOTE

While fitness is the main requirement to pass into the ranks of the SAS, good navigation comes a close second. It is essential that the information detailed on the map be fully recognized and its representation in relation to your route be understood.

best scale to use for cross-country walking is the 1:25,000 Pathfinder map. This larger scale not only shows the rights of way (marked in green), but will also show other useful details such as way-marked routes, camp sites, permissive paths and some areas of open access.

Ordnance Survey maps also show roads, tracks and paths other than those defined as public rights of way. Just because they are shown on the map does not necessarily mean that the public are free to use them. This is clearly stated on the map itself: 'the representation on this map of any other road, track or path is no evidence of the existence of a right of way.' However, in general practice these routes are often travelled along without any hindrance. If the landowners really don't want you there, they will usually put up signs to that effect.

You may notice that some of the lanes and tracks on the map are uncoloured. These 'white roads', as they are sometimes called, often lead to a remote farmhouse or country mansion and as such are normally private. Careful study of the map should give you the answers, but if you are unsure, ask the local authority for advice.

Most maps will give an idea of the 'relief' of an area by showing various heights as contour lines. These are shown as continuous brown lines, with each line defining a certain height (this height will be shown at some point along the line). By studying the contour lines, you will see that as well as showing the height, they also give an idea of the shape of any hill or mountain. If you wish to stay on the level rather than negotiating sharp inclines and declines, use the contours on your map to plan your route. Following a contour where possible is often easier than following a straight line.

MAP SYMBOLS

Map symbols represent objects or places on the ground, for example, a telephone box is marked on the map with capital 'T', while a church with a spire will be represented by a black dot with a cross on top. Rivers and streams are marked in blue with their thickness giving some indication as to size. The routes in this book are normally indicated with a three- or four-figure grid reference which are qualified by the object on the ground. However, not all objects are visibly represented, for example, a trig-point is a man-made fixed concrete object normally on the top of a hill or mountain, while a spot-height only indicates the height of a particular hill above sea level.

Knowing how to use a compass is an essential outdoor skill.

COMPASS

Compasses all work on the principle of having a magnetized needle constantly pointing to North. There are many varieties on the market varying in size and price, but the one most useful for outdoor navigation is the 'Silva'-type compass. This is generally made from clear plastic and is rectangular in shape. The actual compass part is off-set to the left-hand side, while the base contains a magnifying glass and various scales to calculate grid references. The rim of the compass housing can be rotated and is marked with degrees or mil or sometimes both.

As compasses work on the principle of magnetic attraction to the North Pole, it also means that any localized magnetic source will have an effect on your needle; this includes electricity cables, pylons or any heavy metal object. To prevent such sensitivity, some manufacturers line the compass housing with fluid. These often contain a bubble, but as long as it isn't too large, it will not affect the working of the compass.

SETTING A MAP BY INSPECTION

First find a landmark that is both obvious and not likely to disappear overnight; a mountain, river or a road would do the job. Then take a look at your map and find your chosen feature. Once it has been located, simply align the map to the landmark and you will see the other features around you fall into place.

SETTING A MAP BY COMPASS

Lay one of the flat edges of your compass along a North-South grid line on your map. Keeping hold of both the map and the compass, turn both until the needle of the compass is pointing North. Check the surrounding landmarks around you: they should now conform to those on the map.

FINDING A GRID REFERENCE

All maps have grid lines, which are vertical and horizontal thin blue lines superimposed over the terrain. The vertical lines are called 'eastings' because they are numbered from west to east. The horizontal lines are called 'northings' because they are numbered

from south to north. These lines intersect and create squares of a defined area. For example, on a 1:50,000 Landranger map the areas defined by the grid lines are 1 km square.

Obtaining a six-figure grid reference

A grid reference will pinpoint a precise area on the map using both the easting and the northing numbers. The reference of a grid square will consist of four numbers: the first two will be the number shown on the left-hand grid line – the easting – and the second two numbers will be those shown in the middle of the bottom line – the northing. As an example, the grid square in the illustration is 1562. Map references are always given with the easting number first followed by the northing. To find a point within the actual grid square, the square itself is divided up into tenths, so that half way across would be '5'. This number is then added after the relevant easting or northing reference so that an exact point can be located. To work out the tenths precisely, use the romer on your compass, or a protractor. An example of a six-figure grid reference is illustrated above: the location can be read as 155628.

TAKING A COMPASS BEARING FROM THE MAP

A bearing can be defined as the number of degrees in an angle measured clockwise from a fixed northern grid line. Compasses may be marked with 360 degrees, or, more usually, with 6400 mils. Bearings are used to keep you going in the right direction and are especially useful when visibility is bad.

To work out your route, take a good look at the map, noting the terrain, any potential obstacles such as bogs and the distance you will need to travel. Using obvious landmarks, such as a road or a bridge, divide your journey up into easily manageable sections. The point at which you are now, your start-point, should be labelled as 'A' and the landmark at the end of your first section should be labelled point 'B'. To take a bearing from A to B, draw a line between them and place one edge of your compass along it. Be sure that the direction of travel arrow is pointing in the direction you want to go. With the base of the compass held securely in place, rotate the compass dial so that the engraved lines on the dial base lie parallel with the North–South grid lines on the map. Look once more at the direction of travel arrow on the compass housing and read off the bearing next to it. All you will then need to do to use this bearing is to keep the magnetic arrow pointing North over the engraved arrow in the base. You will then be able to follow the direction of travel arrow to point B.

AUTHOR'S TIP

Contouring in fog or bad visibility can produce an interesting effect: most people tend to start wandering downhill. To counter this, make sure you take a few steps in an uphill direction every hundred metres or so. Remember that poor visibility will also mean that you move more slowly.

KEEPING ON COURSE

The direction of your route will depend upon certain factors: the type of terrain has already been mentioned, but the weather and the time of day will also need to be taken into consideration. If you know you will have good weather with good visibility, choose prominent landmarks that can be easily seen both by the naked eye and on the map. Once you have taken your bearing, in the way described above, find an obvious feature in line with the direction you're travelling in and head towards it. With this always in sight, you will not need to check your compass often to make sure that you are keeping on the right route. It will also help you to stay on track if you have to make a slight detour due to some unexpected obstacle. Although a compass is a useful tool, it should not rule you. Always try and keep a mental image of the terrain in your mind, as remembered from the map. With careful route planning and checking landmarks against the map every time you come to one, you should be confident that you will reach your final goal, whatever the weather.

MAGNETIC VARIATION

There are actually three 'Norths' known to science. True North is the fixed location of the North Pole, but this is rarely used for navigational purposes. Grid North is the North depicted on maps by the grid lines. However, Magnetic North is the one most commonly used by those engaged in outdoor pursuits. It is the alignment of the Earth's magnetic field that causes the needle in a compass always to point to Magnetic North. However, every year there are slight changes to the magnetic field and this will also cause the position of Magnetic North to vary. To counteract this, you can use information shown on your map, such as the date it was printed and the degree of variation, to calculate the difference. The result must then be either added to or subtracted from Grid North to obtain an accurate bearing. The way to remember this is:

Mag to Grid = Get Rid
Subtract the variation from your compass bearing before applying it to the map.
Grid to Mag = Add
Add the variation to your map bearing before applying it to your compass.

Although some people insist that calculating this
degree of variation is essential, for most normal
purposes, such as hillwalking, it is hardly necessary. In
fact, over a small distance the difference is just about
negligible anyway. The best solution to this problem is
to shorten the sections of your route, so ensuring that
your bearings still retain a good degree of accuracy.
On the other hand, if you insist on working out the
magnetic variation, bear in mind that it will take you
extra time and there is a high risk that you could
make an error which will throw you completely off
course. Personally, I have never bothered to work out
the magnetic variation unless I have been attempting a
long trek over barren, featureless countryside.

PUTTING A COMPASS BEARING ON THE MAP

Sometimes even the best navigators lose their bearings.
But there is something you can do to relocate your
position on a map by using a compass and a couple of
landmarks. First of all pick out two easily identifiable
features and pinpoint them on your map. Next, take
your compass and point it at the first landmark. Hold
it firmly and turn the housing until the orientating
arrow is aligned with the magnetic needle. Now you
should be able to read off the bearing to the landmark.

To take an example, the bearing to the first landmark
is 5700 mils. If we calculate the magnetic variation,
which, for this example, we'll say is 40 mils, this needs
to be subtracted from the bearing, leaving a revised

figure of 5660 mils. Adjust the compass dial to this amount. On the map, place the top right-hand corner of the compass against the point which represents the landmark and rotate the whole compass until the orienteering lines in the housing are running parallel to the eastings. Draw a line. Repeat the procedure with the second landmark and draw another line. Where the two lines cross is your present position.

GPS (GLOBAL POSITIONING SYSTEM)

This highly technological and modern method of navigation was first developed by the US Department of Defense. There are 24 military satellites orbiting the Earth, constantly transmitting the time and their location. Anyone with a special receiver can pick up this information, whether they are in the military or not. In fact, since GPS systems entered the civilian market their popularity has grown immensely, especially amongst pilots, sailors and walkers. The GPS receiver unit itself is generally no larger than a mobile phone and is powered by battery. It is able to receive and collate the information from the satellites into useful information, such as grid reference and altitude. In fact, you can find out your location no matter where you are in the world. However, there is generally a built-in fault in the civilian units that makes them a little less accurate than the military ones, which can pinpoint a location within 15 metres or less.

How GPS works

For a GPS unit to work, it needs to be able to locate and receive information from at least four of the orbiting satellites, although the more it can pick up, the better. By a process called satellite ranging, the satellite is able to calculate your position in relation to a number of known objects. The transmitted data is then turned into usable information such as longitude and latitude, height above sea level and a grid reference. Your position can be updated, as can your speed and track while on the move. To aid with route planning, it can also identify future way-points. Individual needs can be programmed in, making it flexible whether at sea, on land or in the air.

GPS is state-of-the-art navigation, but always carry a compass as well.

SELECTING A ROUTE

As you are not actually participating in SAS Selection, you have the advantage of choosing your own route. In doing so you can avoid many of the pitfalls which

AUTHOR'S TIP

A GPS unit can be quite costly and will also require a lengthy learning process and plenty of practice before it can be used in a real navigation situation. In the UK the two best models I have come across with regard to instructions are the Silver and the Garmin 40. Even if you do decide to take a GPS unit into the field, bear in mind that it eats batteries and also that the whole system can be shut down at any moment. To this end I advise that you always take a compass as a backup.

lie in wait for the soldiers, such as bogs, rivers, fences and forests. Additionally, you can make your route circular so that you can arrive back at your transport.

The first thing to do is to consult guide books at the local library or talk to a member of the Ramblers' Association. Either of these will give you some information on established walks in your area. If you wish, you can purchase an Ordnance Survey map from which you can select your own route. However, there are several factors to bear in mind.

DISTANCE

The distance of your route should not exceed those examples shown in this book, that is, start off by walking a distance of 5 miles (8 kilometres) and extend this to 10 miles (16 kilometres) as you become more proficient.

TERRAIN

Study the terrain over which you must walk. If you intend leaving a clearly marked footpath and going cross country, make sure you can navigate or read a map and understand the map symbols in the legend. There's nothing wrong with a little hill climbing, but you will find contouring around them much easier. Avoid bogs, crops, thick forests or anything that will bar your way. Do not cross rivers or streams which are more than a foot (30cm) deep.

WAY-POINTS

Way-points are used to guide your path from place to place by establishing a recognizable feature. Clearly

Make your way-points prominent features such as a sharp bend in the road which is recognisable on both the map and the ground.

define the start and finish point of your route. In between make way-points using prominent objects, such as road junctions, bridges and telephone boxes. If you are using a pre-published route card, read and understand the details given. Make sure you know your whereabouts at all points along the route.

TIME AND DISTANCE

Time and distance are both important individual factors, yet your aim should be to bring the two together at a point where you feel most comfortable while achieving the best results. In the initial stages of your exercise programme the time you spend running is far more important than the distance. Get used to running for a certain time and try to increase the distance by simply running faster.

It is best to start off with a minimum time of 30 minutes. Run at a pace you feel comfortable with, which, ideally, should be between 65 to 75 per cent of your heart rate's maximum capacity. If you need to slow down then do so, or if you feel you could do a little more then that's also fine. The important factor at this level is duration, or put another way, time spent increasing the heart rate.

As you improve your running fitness, measure the distance of your routes and time yourself. At this stage simply time yourself while running normally and do not try to set any records.

SAMPLE ROUTES

The following sample routes are designed to help you come to terms with the concept of SAS Selection. You do not have to travel to the Brecon Beacons to walk these routes, moreover you should endeavour to find somewhere near home and select similar routes of your own. Don't forget you are only training and putting into practice all the points mentioned above. Carry a light load (22 lbs (10 kg) max.) and include in this protective clothing, an emergency kit and a light snack. Pace yourself going up hill and jog carefully going downhill to avoid injury. Before you set off leave details of your intended route with someone. The timings shown are based on averaging roughly 16 minutes per kilometre over terrain similar to the Brecon Beacons. The purpose of the following is to help you select and set your own routes, improve your map reading and so prepare you for the extreme fitness programme. While you are encouraged to time your route, finishing is the main goal. I would recommend that you complete no more than two routes per week.

AUTHOR'S NOTE

You should purchase Ordnance Survey map 1:50,000 Landranger Series, Sheet 160 to study the sample route detailed below.

ROUTE 1

This is designed to be a simple map-reading route, starting at one place and finishing at another, and along the way passing through a number of easily recognizable way-points. When selecting a similar route yourself I would advise that you try to avoid difficult or dangerous terrain, and make sure you have a lift waiting for you at the finish.

Route 1

Walking distance: approx. 9 miles (15 km)
Time: 4–5 hours
Dress: equipped for the outdoors; rucksack weight 10 lbs (4.5 kg): warm-up

1 Start at GR896222 where the small track runs southeast from the B-class road. Follow the track as it turns south following it until you are halfway around the forest at Bwleh-y-Duwynt. At this point take a compass bearing on the dam end of Yetradfelle Reservoir, GR945174, and make your own way across country.

2 Upon arrival at Yetradfelle Reservoir take a new bearing heading for the road junction at the southern end of Beacons Reservoir, GR989182.

ROUTE 2

The idea behind Route 2 is to draw a sketch map, which will force you to use your compass, walking from point to point by dead reckoning. This is simply achieved by blotting out the bulk of the map detail leaving just a small patch surrounding each way-point.

Route 2

Walking distance: approx. 11 miles (18 km)
Time: 5–6 hours
Dress: equipped for the outdoors; rucksack weight 10 lbs (4.5 kg); warm-up

1 Start at any of the five points and make your way around them. Each of the areas is in its precise position, making bearings and distance accurate.

2 A: a small road junction at the edge of the forest.

3 B: where a gate leads to a forest track (the stream is not there, but the ground is boggy).

4 C: a river bridge – make sure you get the correct one as there are several near by.

5 D: a river junction in the forest, very easy to find.

6 E: a pool on the edge of a golf course.

My advice is to make your own sketch map using short distances to start with, and then build up to a 5 or 6 kilometres separation. Time and distance are really important, as is recognizing the main feature you are heading for. Sketch maps are designed to aid navigation during poor visibility.

AUTHOR'S TIP

The easiest way to make a sketch map is to place an A4 sheet of paper over the map. Next, using a ten-pence piece, or similar, draw five circles at equal distances apart and cut them out. Lay the paper on top of a map and photocopy and you have one sketch map. Always take a proper map of the area with you, but only use it if you get completely lost.

ROUTE 3

This is the longest route and is designed to test not just your map-reading ability but also your stamina. It uses a main hill feature as the centre point around which the route climbs and descends several times. This helps you concentrate your efforts on improving your overall time.

You should continue practising route planning and map reading until you feel confident enough to participate in the final programme. You will need to have completed at least 10 to 15 such routes before embarking on such a rigorous course.

Route 3

Walking distance: approx. 16 miles (26 km)
Time: 5–8 hours
Dress: equipped for the outdoors; rucksack weight
20 lbs (9 kg); warm-up

1 Start at the car park just south of Cwmgwdi,
   GR024249, which is situated by the old army
   camp. Make your way uphill, heading south-
   southwest, to Twyn Cil-rhew, staying with the
   main track and continuing along the ridge up to
   Pen-y-Fan, GR012215. You can't miss it, it's the
   highest feature in the Beacons range and very
   prominent on a clear day. Be very careful as you
   get close to the top, the northern edge turns into
   a sheer escarpment.

2 From Pen-y-Fan continue walking southwest
   around Corn Du, dropping down the very prominent track to the car park, GR987198 – 1000 m
   south of the Story Arms.

3 Retrace your footsteps back up to Pen-y-Fan turning east at the trig-point 886 dropping down the
   steep slope onto the track that contours south of
   the Graig Cwm Cynwyn ridgeline to point 599,
   GR032205. From here walk directly south along
   Tor Glas until you reach the road/track junction at
   GR035174.

4 Retrace your footsteps back up to Pen-y-Fan, turning north-northeast back down to the car park at Cwmgwdi.

You can do this route from any of the other points, but the Story Arms offers a good starting point as there are toilets and refreshments available – the other locations are accessible but isolated.

SAFETY

If you are new to hillwalking and have no practical knowledge of map reading, I suggest you start by following the more scenic routes, which are clearly

marked and frequently used by other walkers. Almost all the good walks in Great Britain, Europe and America have been well documented in a wide variety of books that are readily available. These will provide a map showing details of the route and will also indicate distance.

Following an established route is a good way to learn map reading.

As with all forms of activity, basic safety rules must be observed. If you intend to walk in an isolated area then any injury or illness that incapacitates you becomes a very serious problem. Therefore you must be prepared.

Safety Precautions

- Whenever possible walk or run your routes in the company of others.

- If alone stick to those routes frequented by others and leave full details of your route and timings with someone trustworthy.

- Carry a mobile phone and have the emergency numbers for the police, rescue services, etc. stuck on the back.

- Always carry a map and compass or route card so that you can indicate your location.

- Dress and carry equipment to suit the prevailing weather conditions.

- Check the weather conditions before you start off.

FINISHING

The aim of these routes is to get fit enough to try out for the SAS Selection. Unlike the SAS soldiers who must complete a given distance in a given time, however, you have no need to rush. Start off by warming up properly and try to avoid routes which go directly into a hill climb. If this is the case, tackle them at a slow pace, keeping your breathing under control. If you start to feel tired, slow down but avoid stopping. If, on the other hand, you feel the need for a little jog along a flat or slight decline then do so. The idea is to reach a point whereby you enjoy walking along, feeling the freedom of the hills and the beauty of nature. When you have completed your route give yourself a little treat: go to the pub with your companions and talk over your accomplishment. Check and note your timings, be critical of any mistakes and praise your efforts. Most of all, relax and soak in the feeling of euphoric fitness.

WARNING

The longest hillwalking exercise described here is six hours, so there is no need to sleep out overnight. However, weather conditions can change quickly and it is wise to take precautions.

SAS TIP

When I was a young soldier in the Welsh Guards there was no such thing as the SFBC; you were simply left to your own devices when it came to getting fit. At the time of volunteering I was stationed in the Middle East. From the start I loaded up a rucksack and ran, and ran, and ran. Lucky for me I was only 22 at the time and my body could take it, but I could easily have over-stretched myself and thus ruined my chances when I arrived at Hereford. But if I learnt anything, it was about running, and running with a bergen.

SAS SELECTION TECHNIQUES

This chapter deals with a series of routes taken while on SAS Selection. If you decide to become super-fit and have prepared yourself properly, you can match your endurance in a similar way to the soldier on SAS Selection. The full programme runs for 17 days, and although soldiers are required to perform non-stop, you have the option of breaking the routes down into a series of weekend activities.

SAS Selection takes place in the Brecon Beacons, South Wales, but as most people will not have access to them they should be used as a guide to make up your own routes. To do this with reasonable accuracy, the area over which you select your routes should be similar in terrain. The Brecon Beacons are not a high range of mountains, but they are treacherous. Exposed and battered by constant weather changes, death by hypothermia is seldom far away for the potential SAS soldiers, and over the years many have suffered this slow death. For the purpose of route selection the British Isles provides many such similar areas to the Brecon Beacons, such as Dartmoor, Snowdonia, the Peak District, Yorkshire Dales and the Lake District. Mid- and North Scotland also provide a whole host of mountainous areas, and all with the added benefit of outstanding scenery.

However, these areas can be equally as dangerous as the Brecon Beacons during bad weather. The build-up training dealt with the basics of good navigation, now we need to know how to equip ourselves properly for walking outdoors.

HILLWALKING EQUIPMENT

Before beginning the next stage of the fitness programme you must make certain preparations. The outdoors can be unpredictable and even dangerous in certain conditions and you will need to ensure that you are properly dressed and equipped. Having the right kind of clothes is especially important to protect the body from the effects of weather. A person's functioning body temperature is usually between 96°F and 102°F. If the body temperature falls outside either of these then vital functions will begin to come under strain and will eventually fail, often leading to death. It is vital that the correct body temperature is maintained, no matter what the weather conditions, otherwise serious complications could occur.

There are many external factors which play a part in affecting the temperature of the body: air temperature; wet; loss of moisture; wind; illness; injury and shock. Body heat can either be leached or added to by the processes of convection, conduction and radiation. However, one of the biggest problems in any outdoor situation is the wind, because it can worsen the situation. If the air temperature is cold and the body wet, the addition of a wind causes an extra chilling factor, taking away vital reserves of body heat and cooling the core temperature of the body too quickly. This will soon cause death. Just as deadly, a wind operating in hot, dry conditions will deplete the body of essential moisture.

Weather can be unpredictable, changing from a hot day to a gale or even a snowstorm within hours. This is especially true in certain climates and also at altitude. Emergencies may occur at any time, so it is always best to be prepared for the worst, so that there is a greater chance that you will survive. In order to protect our body's core temperature you must make sure that you wear the correct protective clothing at all times.

Overheating and excessive sweating will lead to dehydration, causing muscle weakness.

OVERHEATING AND SWEATING

You may be surprised to know that it is possible to get heat exhaustion even when the weather is freezing. This can be caused by exertion while wearing too many layers of clothing. Heat is evenly distributed around the body by the blood, therefore any area in which the bloodflow becomes restricted will soon suffer either from too much heat or not enough. The biggest culprit in restricting bloodflow is tight clothing, especially cuffs around the wrists, ankles, waist and neck. Gloves and socks, too, may cause discomfort and overheating. Always make sure if you're wearing two layers that the outer one is large enough to fit comfortably over the inner one.

At the first sign of overheating act accordingly. Loosen clothing at the neck, wrists and waist to allow a little more air and blood to circulate. If you still find that you're not cooling down enough, start to remove your outer layers of clothing, but do it one layer at a time. Of course, as soon as you stop overheating replace the layers again so that your body does not get chilled. If you need to remove layers when the weather is wet, do not remove any waterproof outer layer, but instead take off one of the inner layers.

The layer system keeps you warm without overheating.

HOW THE LAYER SYSTEM WORKS

One way of controlling body temperature is by using a layer system of clothing. This method depends on lots of thin layers rather than just one or two thick garments. Air gets trapped between the layers and warmed, providing insulation and protection from loss of body heat. The temperature can also be easily controlled by either adding or removing layers.

The clothes that you wear next to your skin should be comfortable, loose-fitting, light and preferably made of a cotton material; for example, a thermal cotton vest would be ideal. As this layer lies closest to the skin it is also the layer which will have to absorb perspiration. It is important, therefore, that under-clothes are changed daily and washed.

Over the top of the underwear you should wear something that, preferably, can be fastened at the neck and wrists. This will further trap any warm air produced by the body. However, the fastenings should not be so tight as to restrict bloodflow. An ideal sort of garment for this would be a sweater with a zip up collar.

The third layer needs to be a warm, easily removable jacket or over-top. Those made from a fleece-type material would be a good choice.

The last layer should always be one that is windproof and waterproof. There are many coats and jackets on the market which are ideal for this purpose. They tend to be made from nylon, fibre-pile material, tightly woven cotton or polycotton. The best outer garments, however, are those made from Gore-Tex as these also allow any trapped condensation to permeate through the material, thus lessening the chances of both chilling and overheating. If possible, always choose a coat with a well-fitting hood so that as much of the face and head can be protected as well.

Remember that any exertion, even fast walking, will cause the body to sweat. This sweat will make your clothing wet and will help leach away body warmth. Sweat, also, over time will cause the fibres of the fabric to deteriorate, thus ruining the clothing.

AUTHOR'S NOTE

If you find yourself getting hot while doing anything strenuous, make sure you remove some of your underlayers. Once you stop your activity, replace them again. By getting into this habit you will ensure that you always have a dry layer next to your skin.

HEAD, HANDS AND FEET

The body loses up to a third of its heat through the head, so this area is of particular importance in both hot and cold climates. Where the weather is cold, it is important to protect this area from heat loss by wearing a scarf or a head-over (a knitted woollen tube worn around the neck and pulled up over the head as required). These items are easy to remove to avoid overheating during strenuous activity. This head protection should still be worn even if your outer garment has a waterproof hood attached.

During hot weather, the body can easily overheat if the head is not covered. Such overheating will lead to sunstroke, which is a potentially fatal condition. An unprotected head also risks serious sunburn. To protect against these possibilities, wear a soft, wide-brimmed hat.

Apart from the head, the other parts of the body to suffer most from the cold and wet are the hands and feet. Both of these are at the extremities of the circulation and therefore liable to suffer a dangerous loss of temperature causing unpleasant and life-threatening conditions, such as frostbite. The best way to prevent this happening is to avoid getting these areas wet and cold in the first place. Feet can be protected by wearing watertight boots and a couple of layers of socks, although it is important that these layers do not impede the circulation at all or else the problem will be made worse. In the same way, ensure that the boots are not too tightly laced. The first sign of the blood-flow being hindered is a feeling of numbness, especially in the toes. Check that this is not happening by stopping every now and again and wriggling your toes. If your feet do happen to get wet, make sure that you change your wet socks for some dry ones at the first opportunity you get.

The hands also need protection. Most gloves are not waterproof and therefore can become very wet. If your hands then become cold as well, they cease to function properly and are a liability to survival as even simple jobs become impossible. If travelling outdoors where cold and wet conditions are a possibility, then you should always carry at least one good pair of loose-fitting gloves with you. The warmest types are mittens as these have a greater amount of air circulating around the fingers, however these are not the most practical if you have to use your fingers a lot to carry out tasks. As well as gloves, it is also a good idea to carry a spare pair of socks as these can also be used instead of gloves if the original pair become too wet to be worn.

Good, comfortable walking boots are essential.

BOOTS AND FOOTWEAR

Feet work hard, covering long distances and supporting your weight, but it is very easy to ignore them – until they start to hurt or get blisters. The way you look after your feet and the type of footwear you choose is more important than you might think if you are contemplating participating in any kind of outdoor activity. Walking, especially if you are carrying a heavy rucksack, puts a great deal of pressure on the feet. In addition you may also be travelling over rough terrain which will subject them to even more stresses. It is common sense that feet and footwear need to be cared for properly.

SELECTING FOOTWEAR

Footwear should always be chosen for the purpose in mind. For the sort of training described in this book a pair of walking boots which combine lightness with adequate ankle support and water protection should be sufficient. There are many boots on the market and the number of styles can be very confusing. To add to the complications, a good pair of boots is usually quite expensive and so most people can only afford one pair at a time. It can often be quite daunting when it comes to choosing the right kind of boot.

Some boots are advertised as being designed for climbing over rugged terrain, while others are better suited to less arduous walks. There are heavy, waterproofed boots for winter conditions, and lighter, cooler ones for the summer. In the end try to find one that provides the best compromise for all of your needs.

Apart from boots, the choice of socks is also important. Heavier boots will need two pairs of socks:

a lightweight inner sock made of wool or silk for warmth, and a thicker outer sock which will act as a cushion for the foot. Lighter boots, made of fabric will need only one pair of socks. There are certain things to consider when buying a new pair of walking boots:

- Take and wear the same kind of socks in which you would normally go walking.

- When your feet are in the boots, your toes should not touch the ends.

- The boot should not feel tight in any area, just comfortable.

- Consider the weight and make sure that it is correct for your needs.

- Choose a boot that is waterproof.

- Make sure that the boot has a well cushioned insole and upper lining, giving firm yet comfortable support to the whole foot.

- The backstay, heel corner and toecap should all be strong enough to protect and support the boot.

AUTHOR'S NOTE

Any foot problems such as corns, bunions or ingrown toenails should be treated before you buy any new footwear.

- The boot should come up high enough around the ankle to give it both support and protection. A padded scree collar and a bellows tongue are also a good idea so that the foot is protected against both water and stones.

- When trying on the boot, stand on an incline; if you feel that your toes are trapped in the end of the boot, try the next size up.

Look at the way the boot was made and consider the maintenance it will need. Fabric boots will not require much more than being kept clean, but leather boots will also need constant applications of wax to keep them supple and watertight. Get a boot with a good grip because this could avoid serious injury, especially if you find yourself on wet and slippery terrain. A rubber star-patterned sole will give you the best grip. PVC will not give much traction at all and is best avoided. Choose a sole thickness in accordance with the sort of terrain you are expecting to walk over. Mountaineering will require a much thicker and stiffer sole than hillwalking. Give the sole a twist to test its flexibility – it should still be solid enough to give good support if you fall.

FOOTWEAR MAINTENANCE

New boots should be worn in before going out on any long walks and this may take some time. It is a small price to pay for comfort, however. Begin by wearing them with the laces a little loose and always check that the tongue is flat against the insole of your foot. Start by going on short walks, or even by wearing them around the house. This will enable you to identify any problems before embarking on a long walk.

The boots will need to be looked after carefully if you want them to last. Clean any mud off as soon as you can before washing them. Once clean, they should be polished or sprayed. Wet leather boots will need to be dried carefully as too much direct heat will cause them to crack. First, take out any detachable insoles and wet laces and dry them separately. Second, stuff

your boots with something absorbent, such as newspaper or tissues and leave them in a warm place. Once the boots have dried they will need to be treated with several applications of wax or some other water-proofing compound.

Choose a rucksack that best suits your walking requirements.

RUCKSACKS

The exercises in this book require that you have a bergen or rucksack large enough to carry all that you need for your walks, as well as items you might need in an emergency situation. These items should include food, water, some kind of shelter, sleeping bag and clothes. Regard your rucksack as a snail would regard its shell: it is your outdoor home, and as such should carry all that you need.

The design of rucksacks has improved remarkably over the years, combining the best of modern technical design and new materials such as two-ply polycotton and Cordura. The rucksacks of today have a high degree of comfort and stability, and come in all shapes and sizes for every kind of outdoor activity. You will need a bergen with a capacity of about 35 litres.

RUCKSACKS AND WEIGHT

Many people who choose their rucksacks wrongly or go for the cheapest options end up with backache, or, even worse, a badly strained back. The spinal column acts as a support for the whole of the upper body, transferring weight down onto the pelvic bones. It is a triumph of engineering in its own right and is constructed as a series of curves which allow for the absorbence of shocks as well as giving the body a good degree of flexibility. The largest of these curves is found in the lower back and is known as the lordosis. This is the part of the spine most designed to take any strain, due to its spring-like construction. Accordingly, this is also the area that is most vulnerable to backache.

When choosing a rucksack bear the above in mind and make sure that it fits in with your body shape, preferably with a wide, padded waistbelt as this will take some of the weight off the spine and transfer it straight to the hips. The centre of gravity of the pack should be high on your back, with the rest of the weight evenly distributed between your shoulders and your hips. This will ensure that instead of the back doing all the work, your legs will also help to bear the weight. When the rucksack is full, make sure that it is able to support the weight in a stable manner.

FITTING YOUR PACK

Packing a rucksack correctly is an art and one that should be learned before you go out into the field. First, you need to know what to pack so that unnecessary items are left at home, not adding to the weight on your back. Second, you should be sure that once everything is packed you can still get at anything you want with a minimum of effort.

Side pockets are the easiest to get to and therefore should hold things you will need while you are walking, such as water, flasks and snacks. These pockets are also useful for carrying Camel hydration systems (a tube and water container set-up that allows the walker to drink without having to stop). Coats and items of clothing needed if the weather turns nasty should be neatly folded beneath the top flap of your rucksack. The bergen itself should be packed with items used less frequently, such as a sleeping bag, at the bottom, and those you are likely to use more often at the top.

SAS TIP

Sometimes in the SAS it seems that you are forever walking attached to your bergen. This seems to start with Selection and then continues throughout your service. Therefore if anyone knows how to pack a bergen, an SAS soldier does. Before every operation he will scrutinize the contents of his pack, taking out anything that will be unnecessary and therefore add to the weight. This also sometimes means a bit of improvisation: throwing away any excess food wrappings and even taking food out of tins and repackaging it in plastic bags. Luxuries are a complete non-starter. When it comes down to it, you should be able to put your rucksack on your back and then forget about it as you walk. If it is too heavy or unbalanced, this will not be possible and you will find the walk an awful experience.

SAS SELECTION ROUTES.

The following 18-day fitness course is designed around the early exercise tests encountered while doing SAS Selection. However, in addition to their rucksacks the participating soldiers will be expected to carry a rifle and a 15-lb (7-kg) belt kit. The sample routes are based on those covered by the SAS and should be used as a guide to plan similar routes in your chosen area.

Food consumption during this 18-day course is unlimited with the suggestion that you plan a high protein and carbohydrate diet. Not that you will feel like drinking alcohol but you should abstain altogether during the course.

The course has two sets of rest days spaced at five-day intervals. You should use the rest days to relax, treat any medical problems, eat and sleep.

Day One

Dress: equipped for outdoors
Rucksack weight: 30 lbs (14 kg)

Morning:
Warm-up. Find a suitable road and complete the following fitness test. You will need a friend to assist you in some of the exercises.

5-km run; fireman's lift 100 m; 20 push-ups;
baby carry 200 m; 2-mile walk

Afternoon:
Find a steep hill of at 100 m.
Warm-up, then complete 20 x 100 m up the hill.
No time limit.

Day Two

Dress: equipped for outdoors
Rucksack weight: 40 lbs (18 kg)

Fan Dance

Warm-up. Find a mountainous peak of around 1000
m above sea level and choose three points around
the peak at a distance of around 3 miles
(5 km). Total distance 15 miles (24 km).
Sample route:

Start-point lay-by grid 987198 ➤ RV1 Pen-y-Fan grid 012 216 ➤
RV2 Track junction 033 182 ➤ RV3 Pen-y-Fan grid 012 216 ➤
RV4 Road / bridge junction grid 985241 ➤ RV5 Pen-y-Fan grid
012 216 ➤ finish-/start-point grid 987198

Complete the distance inside 6 hours.

Day Three

Dress: equipped for outdoors
Rucksack weight: no rucksack required

Beasting

Warm-up. Find a short flat deserted road or track. You
will require the services of a friend about your own
weight. Complete the following in under 1 hour:

Firemans-lift 200m; 20 push-ups; baby carry 200m; 20 push-
ups; piggy-back ride 200m; 20 push-ups; fireman's lift 200m;
20 push-ups; baby carry 200m; 20 push-ups; piggy-back 200m;
20 push-ups.

Afternoon:

Locate a steep hill of at least 200 metres. Warm-up. Complete
20 x 200 m up the hill.

Day Four

Dress: equipped for outdoors
Rucksack weight: 40 lbs (18 kg)

Warm-up. Swimming test: 20 circuits of the local swimming pool. Tread water for 10 minutes.
Afternoon:
Map-reading exercise: sample route – start-point road/lay-by grid 0175 1060 ➤ RV1 bridge grid 9450 1120 ➤ RV2 pot-hole grid 8910 1615 ➤ finish-point road junction grid 844 164.
No time limit.

Days Five and Six

Rest days.

Day Seven

Dress: equipped for outdoors
Rucksack weight: 30 lbs (14 kg)

Warm-up. Map-reading exercise number 2: choose a hilly area some 11 miles (18 km) in distance.
Sample route – start-point road/stream junction grid 967126 ➤ RV1 Yetradfelle reservoir grid 944 073 ➤ RV2 road/stream junction grid 926208 ➤ finish-point lay-by grid 855179.
Time taken 5hours.

Day Eight

Dress: equipped for outdoors
Rucksack weight: 40 lbs (18 kg)

Warm-up. Map-reading exercise number 3: choose a route about 9 miles (15 km) in distance over lowland forested terrain. Sample route: start-point road junction grid 1080 6465 ➤ RV1 trig-point 538 grid 1705 6065 ➤ RV2 east end of pool grid 1400 5940 ➤ RV3 telephone box grid 1255 5820 ➤ finish-point road/river bridge grid 1140 5445
Time taken 4hours 30 minutes.

Day Nine

Dress: equipped for outdoors
Rucksack weight: 40 lbs (18 kg)

Warm-up. Map-reading exercise number 4: choose a route about 12 miles (20 km) in distance over lowland forested terrain. Sample route: start-point pub car park grid 8810 2915 ➤ RV1 standing stones grid 8335 2835 ➤ RV2 standing stones grid 8360 2570 ➤ RV3 spot-height 591 grid 8475 2315 ➤ RV4 spot-height 562 grid 8620 2065 ➤ RV5 spot-height 582 grid 9080 2640 ➤ finish-/start-point grid 8810 2915
Time taken 4hours 30 minutes.

Day Ten

Dress: equipped for outdoors
Rucksack weight: 40 lbs (18 kg)

Warm-up. Map-reading exercise number 5: choose a route about 8½ miles (14 km) in distance over hill and forested terrain. Sample route: start-point telephone box grid 172 585 ➤ RV1 spot-height 523 grid 193 609 ➤ RV2 trig-point 660 grid 182 639 ➤ RV3 spot-height 491 grid 159 635 ➤ RV4 trig-point 538 grid 171 606 ➤ finish-/start-point grid 172 585
Time taken 4 hours.

Day Eleven

Dress: equipped for outdoors
Rucksack weight: 45 lbs (20 kg)

Warm-up. Map reading exercise number 6: choose a route about 18 miles (29 km) in distance over mixed hill and forested terrain. Sample route: start-point road junction grid 160 647 ➤ RV1 spot-height 491 grid 159 635 ➤ RV2 AA box grid 198 598 ➤ RV3 trig-point 610 grid 214 636 ➤ RV4 stream junction grid 202 671 ➤ Finish-/start-point grid 160 647
Time taken 6 hours.

Days Twelve and Thirteen

Rest days.

Day Fourteen

Dress: equipped for outdoors
Rucksack weight: 50 lbs (23 kg)

Pipeline

Warm-up. Choose a route about 14 miles (23 km) in distance over steep hills. Sample route: start-point lay-by near dam grid 987 198 ➤ RV1 spot-height 632 grid 938 186 ➤ RV2 pot-hole grid 891 161 ➤ RV3 trig-point 725 grid 881 191 ➤ RV4 trig-point 603 grid 912 216 ➤ RV5 spot-height 632 grid 938 186 ➤ finish-/start-point grid 987 198.
Time taken 5 hours 30 minutes

Day Fifteen

Dress: equipped for outdoors
Rucksack weight: 50 lbs (23 kg)

Point to Point

Choose a route about 25 km in distance over steep hills. Sample route: start-point lay-by grid 972 222 ➤ RV1 Pen-y-Fan grid 012 216 ➤ RV2 car park grid 024 249 ➤ RV3 Pen-y-Fan grid 012 216 ➤ RV4 track junction grid 034 182 ➤ RV5 Pen-y-Fan grid 012 216 ➤ finish-/start-point grid 972 222
Time taken 6 hours.

Day Sixteen

Dress: equipped for outdoors
Rucksack weight: 70 lbs (32 kg)

Heavy Carry
Choose a route about 9 miles (15 km) in distance over steep hills. Sample route: start-point road junction grid 773 259 ➤ RV1 stone circle grid 808 244 ➤ RV2 trig-point 802 grid 826 218 ➤ finish-point road junction grid 861 246
Time 4 hours 30 minutes.

Day Seventeen

Dress: equipped for outdoors
Rucksack weight: 55 lbs (25 kg)

Endurance
Choose a route about 40 miles (65 km) in distance over steep hills. Sample route: start-point road junction grid 080 260 ➤ RV1 track junction grid 034 182 ➤ RV2 Fan Fawr grod 964 189 ➤ RV3 trig-point 603 grid 912 216 ➤ RV4 road / track junction grid 868 193 ➤ RV5 Yetradfelle reservoir grid 944 073 ➤ RV6 road bridge grid 995 164 ➤ RV7 track junction grid 034 183 ➤ finish-point grid 080 260
Time taken 20 hours.

Complete the course within the times and you should be proud of yourself. Completion within an hour of the times is also good and still gives you something to aim for.

FITNESS HEALTH AND INJURIES

AVOIDING INJURY

A medical chapter in a fitness book may at first seem strange, but the reasons for its inclusion will soon become apparent. For a start it serves as a warning not to exercise while overweight or seriously unfit. This can damage a body that is unused to exertion. In the worst case it could lead to a heart attack. Even in a fit person, exercise can still cause injury if that person is not careful about the way he uses his body.

This chapter aims to focus on the risks and medical problems associated with getting fit and exploring the great outdoors. It is one thing getting a sprain or blisters either at home or in the gym, but if you sustain the same injury while walking out alone in remote areas with the weather closing in, it could be a matter of life and death. This is not to say that the potential dangers should put you off: the advantages of exercising still far outweigh any risks. However, there is nothing wrong with being aware that something might just go awry, and knowing what you can do about it. It is wise to be prepared.

Intense exercising will often cause injuries as the body is pushed beyond its normal limits. However, with a sensible training regime it should be possible to minimize any risk and stay safe. A well-balanced exercise programme will always include a warm-up and cool down, will never place too much stress on any one part of the body, and will allow time for recovery. If any part of your body has a weakness, start off by strengthening it with gentle exercises; stretching will limit the possibility of damage. Run or jog on a smooth, level surface to avoid sprains and strains. Bear in mind that most problems are caused by overusing a muscle or a joint, exercising too much or too intensely without time for the body to recover.

If, despite taking every precaution, you find that you have injured yourself, stop what you are doing immediately and seek medical help. Carrying on will only make it worse, whereas an injury that is treated straight away will stand a better chance of healing quickly. Most injuries caused by overuse can be treated with RICE – rest, ice, compression and elevation. Injuries are generally caused by:

- Being overweight or too unfit while exercising.
- Training too hard and too quickly.
- Playing in a high-contact sport such as rugby.
- Hard surfaces.
- Addiction to exercise (where it becomes the be-all and end-all of your life).
- Traffic accidents (this applies mainly to roadrunners and cyclists).

TRAINING WHILE UNFIT OR OVERWEIGHT

This subject has been well covered, however, it is wise to remember the repercussions. Pushing you body into a series of strenuous exercises while grossly overweight or unfit can and most likely will produce a heart attack. The only way to approach fitness safely is to lose weight and exercise slowly. Apart from physical injury, such as a strain or broken bone, you should also be aware of other symptoms during exercise. These symptoms include:

- Severe chest pain
- Sudden headache
- Abdominal pain
- Dizziness
- Nausea and vomiting
- Severe pain to the body without obvious physical reason

Always take prompt action. Stop exercising and rest. If the symptoms continue or reoccur after exercise is resumed then you should seek immediate medical assistance.

TRAINING TOO HARD

While enthusiasm is a great motivator, exercising beyond your current physical condition will only produce a negative affect. As any marathon runner will tell you, there is a point at which the body is totally drained of energy; to exercise beyond this point will cause muscle fatigue. Always exercise so that the body's aerobic system is functioning at around 75–80 per cent of capacity.

Contact sports invariably cause injury.

CONTACT INJURIES

We are not all inclined to take up walking as a form of fitness. Some people prefer more social sports such as football, martial arts or bike riding. The problem here is contact. Contact when tackled by another player, contact when your opponent hits you with a miss-guided punch, or when a dog runs in front of you and you fall off your bike, making contact with the road.

TRAFFIC ACCIDENTS

Accidents on the road involving joggers and cyclists are not that frequent but can be very serious. Avoidance is the best defence against a road traffic accident. Jog or walk on tracks not used by vehicles. Don't wear headphones while running on the road.

Wear light or reflective clothing during the hours of dusk and darkness.

TRAINING ON A HARD SURFACE

Running on hard surfaces causes many leg injuries, especially in the knee. Avoid running on hard road surfaces or concrete. Soft, even surfaces are best for injury prevention. Whenever possible, run on grass or dirt paths, or in parks. However, if hard surface running is all that is available to you, make sure you exercise with appropriate footwear for the conditions, and allow extra recovery periods.

To avoid the risk of injury, don't jog or run on a hard surface.

FITNESS OBSESSION

It must be stressed that all forms of training and exercising must be done at a set pace and in balance with the body's resources. If you push yourself too hard for too long, you will begin to feel fatigued. Overtraining will do very little to improve your fitness.

If anything, it will cause your body to become listless or even to shutdown. The main symptoms of fatigue are a sharp decrease in energy and stamina followed by flu-like symptoms and increased weight loss.

Recovery from exercise fatigue is total rest and an increased diet. All forms of fitness should be suspended until your appetite has fully returned and the body has reverted to its normal balance. Stress and poor diet will only prolong the fatigue.

SAS TIP

An ex-military friend of mine who is now employed as a gym teacher set himself the goal of running a 5-day marathon across the Saudi Arabian desert. At the age of 59 this would have been a major achievement. He trained exceptionally hard – too hard. On the fourth day of the race he became sluggish and floundered, unable to carry on. He had pushed himself too hard during training. Upon his return to England he was a different man, fatigue had set in which had totally demoralized him.

TYPICAL INJURIES

Certain injuries are more commonly associated with exercise than others. These are:

- Chafing (abrasions caused either by skin rubbing against skin or material rubbing against skin)

- Broken bones, dislocations or displacement of one or more bones in a joint
- Blisters
- Sprains and muscle strains
- Back injuries
- Shinsplints

SHINSPLINTS

These are injuries caused to the shinbones and the soft tissues in that area. They are generally caused by running on hard surfaces without good shock protection or wearing shoes with rigid soles. Running or walking on the balls of the feet will also cause this painful injury.

YOUR FEET

Without feet many of the exercises in this book, such as the hillwalking, jogging and running, could not be done. That is why it is so important that the feet are cared for. For instance, ingrown toenails and blisters should be treated as soon as they occur, otherwise they will only get more painful and end up delaying or even preventing you continuing with the exercise programme.

BLISTERS

Blisters on a foot are something that most people have experienced at some time in their life. They are usually caused by footwear that doesn't fit properly, socks of poor quality or loose laces. In addition to these, having to walk long distances over rough terrain, especially if the foot becomes wet, will cause blisters to develop.

In general, blisters are not serious and can be treated as a minor injury. However, the pain they cause can often be so bad as to be disabling and this will be disastrous if out on a long walk and a good way from home. To avoid getting blisters, make sure that your footwear fits well and is well worn in before attempting any long excursions. Also, make sure that your feet are kept clean and dry.

Serious blisters can be avoided if treated immediately.

Blisters should be treated the moment they appear; to leave them longer will create a sore that may become infected and slow to heal. As soon as you feel a sore spot, stop, put some antiseptic cream on it and cover it with a plaster or a surgical dressing, making sure there are no creases in the tape. Micropore tape can be used on the toes. If a fluid-filled blister is already present, use a blister ring instead. This will protect the area against any further pressure.

A large fluid-filled blister will often be extremely uncomfortable. The pressure can be relieved by draining the fluid. Do not do this by bursting it, as this will only expose an area of raw skin underneath and leave it open to infection. Wash the foot thoroughly first and then sterilize a needle. Prick the blister at the bottom edge and then gently press out the fluid, taking as much time as it needs. Once this has been done, cover the area with a blister ring. This should be changed every day and the area cleansed each time. Blisters can be helped to heal by immersing the foot in a hot, salty footbath. However, make sure that you dry off the area around the blister thoroughly – blisters need to be clean and dry to heal.

INGROWN TOENAILS

Ingrown toenails are painful enough to prevent exercise, and should be treated as soon as they are

detected. Cutting a 'V' down the centre of the nail will help relieve the pain. However, if the toe has become infected you are advised to see a chiropodist or your doctor for treatment at once, because the nail will most probably need removing.

SAS TIP

One survival method of relieving the pressure from an ingrown toenail is to shave the top centre of the nail with a safety razor blade. Skim the middle third of the nail, shaving from the bed towards the nail-tip. Place a thin piece of plastic under the nail to prevent any accidental cutting of the toe front. When the nail is thin enough it will buckle into a ridge and relieve the outer pressure. Removing the nail altogether should be avoided, as this will require a dressing and may prevent exercise for several weeks.

SPRAINS

Sprains happen when a joint is pushed beyond its normal limitations of movement. The ligaments supporting the joint become overstretched and some of the fibres may even tear. However, they do not break completely and the structure of the joint remains, for the most part, intact. Sprains are extremely painful and will cause swelling and some-times even a haematoma around the area affected. The joint becomes severely weakened, losing its ability to support weight, and sometimes even its ability to move. Because of these symptoms, severe sprains are often confused with having broken a bone. In cases like these, the only way to be sure is to get to a hospital and have an X-ray. Very severe sprains or injuries in which the ligaments have been completely torn will require hospital treatment, which usually involves the injured part being operated on, splinted or put in a cast.

Less severe sprains should immediately be treated by rest, ice, compression and elevation. You should rest the injured part in an elevated position and apply a cold compress – a bag of frozen peas, for example, wrapped in a towel is ideal. Then tape the injury, but not too tightly, to inhibit further swelling. Once the swelling has decreased, usually about after 24 hours, heat can then be applied to relieve any pain and to help the circulation.

CRAMP

Cramp is an extremely painful but luckily not a particularly serious condition which doesn't usually last for very long. It occurs when a muscle (or muscles) suddenly goes into an involuntary contraction, becoming hard and rigid. Cramps can affect any muscle but most commonly occur in the calf muscles and seem to happen either when at rest after strenuous exercise, or at night. Any activity that makes you sweat, or any activity undertaken in hot weather will increase your chance of getting a cramp due to the loss of salt and water in the body. Usually the pain disappears within a few minutes and until then a certain amount of relief can be gained by gently massaging the area.

Chafing can be prevented and treated by a liberal application of petroleum jelly.

CHAFING

Chafing is caused by friction against the skin. This can be due either to material or else contact with another area of skin. It is usually experienced either in the armpits, the groin or on the nipples, and in the worst cases can be very painful. The material of a vest or T-shirt rubbing constantly against the sensitive area can cause chafing of the nipple. To stop it, change your vest or T-shirt to one with softer material and use Vaseline as a lubricant. If you are a long way from home and it is becoming unbearable, rip a small hole out of the material in the nipple area.

Chafing of the armpits or the groin is usually caused by the rubbing of skin against skin, especially during a repeated movement, although clothing can also cause friction here too. As before, the remedy is a good application of petroleum jelly, but make sure that you apply it before you exercise. If you let the chafing continue without treatment, not only will it become very sore, but it may also become infected, which would disrupt your exercise programme.

RUCKSACK ABRASION

Rucksacks can produce sore spots or abrasions on the back and shoulders if they are badly fitted, badly packed, too heavy or poorly padded. The common areas where abrasions occur are the shoulders, waist (around the kidney area) and the lower back. First of all, always choose a rucksack that fits your body properly, that way you should be able to shoulder the pack for the whole of your route without really feeling it. If at any point you feel any abrasions beginning to develop, try and adjust the straps so that the pack sits better on your back and shoulders. If this doesn't help, identify where the abrasions are at their worst and add extra padding of some kind. Use petroleum jelly to ease the friction and soothe any soreness.

NATURAL HAZARDS

Many people underestimate the dangers present in nature. Any trek off the beaten track will need thorough preparation so that you will know what to do if you get into any difficulties. The first thing to be aware of is the weather: it can change without warning from a beautiful sunny day to cold rain, snow or fog. Fog, in particular, will cause a rapid decline in visibility which can leave you lost and disorientated. Secondly, terrain can cause problems: rocky ground or rivers can be dangerous, and a walk in the mountains may prove to be more arduous than first thought. Injuries, or even illness, can occur without warning and you may be in a remote place where you will be unable to summon help.

TRAINING ALONE

To be safe, never go it alone in any isolated area, no matter how much you love the solitude. A walking partner could prove invaluable in times of difficulty, especially if you sustain a life-threatening injury or become unconscious. Make sure that you are properly dressed and equipped. Make sure that your footwear is up to the job and that your rucksack carries camping equipment. Make sure, also, that you are physically able to do the trip. A good knowledge of first aid could prove invaluable in an emergency.

Despite the above advice there will still be people who will insist on walking alone. If you are one of these, it is essential to follow a few simple rules:

- Always leave a copy of your route and an estimated time you can be expected back. Leave this with someone you know to be responsible.

- Consider taking your mobile phone along. Although they don't work in many remote areas, some mountainous places will have radio relays on top of them. Make sure you have the numbers of the rescue services programmed into the phone or taped onto the back. In an accident, this could save your life.

DEHYDRATION

Water makes up the largest proportion of our bodies – around 75 per cent. It is essential to the proper functioning of the body that it is kept at this level. Problems will start when about two pints are lost and if this isn't replaced the more serious condition of heatstroke will occur, which can lead to death.

Dehydration occurs when bodily fluid lost through perspiration, breathing, urination and excretion is not replaced. Therefore it is essential to drink when undertaking any form of exercise that causes excessive sweating, or if the weather is hot.

To reduce the risk of fluid loss, especially if you do not have access to plentiful supplies of good drinking water, you will need to conserve the water already in your body. Make sure that you cover up any exposed skin: not only will this help retain water, it will also protect you against sunburn. Rest as much as possible in the hottest part of the day and limit any activity. Try and find shelter, or attempt to build yourself a basic one. Finally, avoid smoking or drinking alcohol as this will only serve to dehydrate you further.

HEAT EXHAUSTION

Heat exhaustion or heatstroke is a potentially serious condition caused when the body overheats. This can easily happen if you are exerting yourself in hot, dry conditions. The symptoms are weakness and dizziness, the skin may be cold and clammy to touch. Immediate treatment is to get into some shade and rest. The body needs to be cooled as quickly as possible. Make sure clothing is loosened so that air can circulate and pour some cold water over the head and neck. Any lost fluid must be replaced by drinks of water, if possible with a little salt added. Rest is recommended until recovery takes place, but then things must be taken very slowly or else it could happen again.

SALT

An average human body needs 10 gms of salt a day to help it function; if the levels fall below this, problems will result. Salt is next in importance to water as it helps to control the homeostasis of the body. Sweating can cause a depletion of salt in the body as sweat contains salt as well as water. Salt deficiency is characterized by muscle cramps, nausea, weakness and a hot, dry sensation in the body. As with heatstroke, at the first sign of salt depletion rest in the shade and drink a mug of water, to which has been added a small pinch of salt. If you feel salt loss and dehydration might be a problem on your trip, carry a couple of sachets of rehydration powder in your first-aid kit.

COLD

Exposure to the cold can be deadly. Temperatures below freezing combined with wet and wind create the perfect conditions for hypothermia or frostbite to strike. Wind, in particular, has a severe effect on temperature because the cooling effects of cold air are increased by its movement. This is known as wind chill. For example, air moving at 30 mph (48 km/h) and having a temperature of -20°C (-4°F) has the same chilling effect as air at -40°C (-104°F) moving at only 5 mph (8 km/h). If the weather is wet as well, this will make matters worse as water will help to remove heat from the body. Wet clothes lose their insulating properties.

To combat the threat of hypothermia, use the layer system of clothing as detailed on page 137, as this will help to trap more warm air close to your body and can also be adjusted to avoid sweating. Sweating needs to be avoided because, like rain, it will reduce the insulation levels of your clothes and conduct your body heat away to the out-side. It will also cool the skin. Remember: do everything you can to keep dry, and if your clothes do get wet, either dry them, or get into some dry ones as soon as possible.

Both wet cold and dry cold can cause hypothermia. Even SAS soldiers have died due to a lack of adequate protection from the elements.

Hands and feet, in particular, need to be looked after in the cold. They are the parts that receive the circulation last and are therefore the first to lose it when they get too cold. Make sure that you do not restrict the bloodflow to them by having fastenings at the wrists and ankles too tight, and keep them dry as much as you can. Be aware of any signs of numbness and keep the parts moving. If you need to warm your hands, do so under your armpits or between your thighs. Feet can be kept warm by wriggling the toes, although if they have slight frostbite they can be warmed against a companion. If there are no serious signs, give them a gentle massage. Do not, however, expose any frost-nipped parts to direct heat.

Always carry a spare pair of socks to change into in case yours become wet. In any case, a change of socks once a day will keep your feet in good, hygienic condition. Every now and again, take your boots and socks off and give your feet a massage for about ten minutes. Plastic bags placed over walking boots will add extra insulation, but be careful not to slip.

HYPOTHERMIA

Once body temperature falls below 35°C (95°F), the body starts to suffer from hypothermia. With body heat being lost faster than it can be replaced, the organs of the body begin to slow down until, if nothing is done, death occurs. You are at most danger of hypothermia when you are cold, wet, tired, injured or ill. Conditions such as inadequate clothing, immersion in cold water and a lack of food or drink will all exacerbate this condition. The symptoms come on very gradually, so it is not always easily diagnosed. However, you will need to be aware if you, or anyone else, are subject to the following:

- Uncontrollable shivering
- Pale, dry skin which is sub-normally cold to the touch
- Muscular weakness and tiredness
- Apathy
- Irrational behaviour
- Change in personality; for example, a quiet person may become aggressive
- Eyesight failing
- The need to sleep
- Slow, weak pulse
- Slow, shallow breathing
- Eventual collapse and unconsciousness; possible cardiac arrest

At the first suspicion of hypothermia, everything possible must be done to restore the lost body heat. The casualty needs to rest, out of the cold and wet. Get into some type of shelter if possible, or construct a simple one out of whatever materials are to hand. Wet clothes need to be replaced with dry ones as soon as possible as they will reduce the body heat further. This is particularly important if the casualty has been submerged in water. All clothing in this case will need to be removed as these will kill the sufferer quicker than by just being naked.

Hypothermia is a killer and should be treated immediately.

The casualty can be warmed in a variety of ways. If she is conscious, and you have the means, get her to eat or drink something hot. Those who constantly exercise outdoors should carry a metallized survival blanket, which is wonderful for warming a hypothermia victim. These blankets are certainly worth considering as they hardly take up any room in your rucksack and yet can be lifesavers. If another healthy person is present, they will also be able to help warm the casualty by sharing their own body heat.

When hypothermia reaches a certain stage, the casualty may become unconscious. If there are no signs of breathing or a pulse, start resuscitation techniques immediately, but don't neglect to keep the sufferer warm. Resuscitation should still be undertaken even if the body temperature has fallen below 26°C (78.8°F), which is when death usually occurs. Even at this stage you cannot assume they are dead and give up. Use assisted ventilation and chest compressions until the body's temperature gets back to normal. If you still cannot revive her after that then she is most likely dead.

Any casualty suffering from either hypothermia or frostbite will need to be handled very carefully, because frozen skin and flesh are extremely delicate and prone to damage. There are several things you can do that will help, as well as certain things that will cause further damage:

- Provide shelter from the wind and cold as soon as possible.
- Do not rub or massage to stimulate circulation.
- Do not warm the casualty by using external fire or heat.
- Give hot food or drink if the casualty is conscious. Chocolate and other high-calorie foods are also good.
- Do not allow the casualty to drink alcohol.
- The casualty must not exert himself in anyway.
- If dry clothing or covering is available, use it to replace any wet clothing.

If it is necessary to replace wet clothing, it should be done piece by piece so that only one part of the body is uncovered at any one time. If you do not have any spare dry clothing, but do have a sleeping or a survival bag, leave the casualty in her wet clothes and place her in the bag. Make sure that it is both windproof and waterproof and that it will retain or reflect body heat. This will ensure that the casualty will not lose any more heat, and, at the very least, will stay stable. If another healthy person is available, they can help by sharing the same survival bag and giving some of their body heat to the casualty.

AUTHOR'S NOTE

Hypothermia strikes quickly and without warning during wet, windy and cold conditions. Many hill-walkers and even experienced SAS soldiers have met their deaths through not recognizing it or not being able to treat it early on. I cannot emphasize enough the importance of being aware of hypothermia and the danger it presents.

CALORIE-COUNTED MENUS AND FOODS

For most people eating is one of the most pleasurable facets of human life. However, when we are dieting or participating in excessive exercise our food demands differ. If we are dieting then our goal is to reduce body fat. We have seen in the previous chapters that restricting calorie intake while increasing exercise activity does this. At the other end of the scale participating in excessive exercise demands a higher calorie intake to maintain the body's nutritional balance. Although we deal with both situations separately, there are only two rules that should always be adhered to: always eat a wide range of foods; and keep to your daily calorie allowance. By doing so you will ensure an adequate intake of all the body's nutritional requirements.

DIET CONTROL

If we are honest with ourselves, no-one really enjoys dieting, nevertheless for some of us it is a necessity. Yet there is no reason why the limited food we consume should be boring. All food should be pleasurable to the palate and well presented. Avoid an all fruit and vegetable diet because of the high water content which eventually can lead to malnutrition. Additionally, the body will need some fat.

It is not within the scope of this book to detail a whole host of menus, but to get you started I have outlined some sample menus which are listed below. As we all enjoy different tastes it is up to the you what you actually consume and the range of low-calorie meals is only limited by your imagination. When you eat take time to savour the taste and try to avoid rushed meals. A few simple tips will help reduce the calorie intake and still provide an appetizing meal:

- Reduce portions or bulk out with low-calorie foods.
- Drink water or low-calorie drinks.
- Avoid sugar-rich sauces, use reduced fat dressings.
- Use skimmed milk.
- Boil or poach foods, rather than grill or fry.
- Substitute sugar with sweeteners.
- Reduce salt intake.
- Avoid alcohol with meals.

Your diet can be helped by restricting the calorie count according to meal type. For example, breakfast 300, lunch 300, dinner 600, drinks 300; total intake 1500 calories. An example of this would be:

- Breakfast: fresh orange juice, poached egg on wholemeal toast.
- Lunch: tuna sandwich, bottle of spring water and apple.

- Dinner: Fitness Stew, low-calorie flan, glass of spring water.
- Drinks: 1½ Pints of beer or 2 small tots of spirits

PREPARE YOUR OWN FOOD

The reason for preparing your own food is firstly you control the amount and secondly you control the preparation and the ingredients. The volume of food we eat will depend on what weight loss we are trying to achieve and the type of food being prepared. In using food volume to control weight loss one must be careful that you do not under-eat and deprive your body of vital nutrients and vitamins. The type of food being prepared is also important, meats are generally high in protein where vegetables are not. We must also take into consideration ingredients such as cooking oils, dressing, sources, salt and other additives. Wherever possible use fresh produce. Choose lean meat and healthy looking vegetables and fruit, if fresh is not available use frozen. Avoid eating prepacked, prepared or tinned meals when on a diet, they contain too many preservatives.

Salad can be eaten as a main meal or to bulk out a small portion of high-protein food.

BULKING MEALS WITH VEGETABLES

Although supplying the required calorific value, many diets lack substance, especially when it comes to appearances and size. The restaurant trade found the ideal solution to this many years ago – add lots of colourful salad. Not only does this brighten the appearance but is also bulks out the meal while adding minimal food value.

Eating salad as a main meal is also a good idea, though the appearance somehow lacks body. One way around this problem is to convert you plain salad into a sort of ploughman's lunch or a Greek *mese*. Its easy to get carried away with the amount of relish, cheese, taramasalata and humus so try to keep these to a minimum and improve the salad by adding pickled onions, beetroot and tuna fish.

FRUIT

The benefits of eating one or two portions of fruit each day are enormous. Fruit contains hardly any saturated fats and is rich in fibre. Added to breakfast cereals it helps take away the taste of eating all those dry and unpalatable bran flakes, and it makes a great snack if you are feeling hungry or just peckish between meals.

Best Meal: mixed fruit salad is an excellent meal, either for breakfast or as a dessert after your main meal (10½-oz (300-g) portion is around 150 calories).

BREAD

Despite what other diet books say, and provided you
stay within the recommended daily intake (3 slices
while dieting, 6 slices normal), bread is a versatile
food platform. Almost everyone over the age of two
eats some bread every day, either with a meal (bulk-
ing) or as a sandwich snack. It can accompany every
kind of food – salad, vegetables, meat, cheese, jam and
so on. A large (British) slice of bread is around 80
calories for wholemeal and 110 for white. The
following sandwiches are a guide based on two slices
of wholemeal bread spread lightly with polyunsaturat-
ed margarine. If you want to liven up your sandwich
use pickles, which average around 130 calories per
3½ oz (100 g) opposed to mayonnaise which contains
some 700 plus calories.

Sample Sandwiches

Beetroot sandwich = 258 calories
Boiled egg sandwich = 377 calories
Cottage Cheese and tomato sandwich = 290 calories
Ham sandwich = 320 calories
Strawberry jam sandwich = 350 calories
Bacon sandwich = 690 calories
Corned beef sandwich = 437 calories
Chicken sandwich = 348 calories
Tuna sandwich = 290 calories

EGGS

While eggs are full of saturated fats, they are also full of goodness. A single boiled/poached egg is around 120 calories and with a slice of toast it makes a tasty and filling breakfast. It is best to restrict your egg intake to a maximum of four eggs per week, while taking part in any dietary programme, and six per week under normal conditions.

Best Meal: pick a small bowl of fresh nettle leaves and boil for about 20 minutes (substitute spinach if you can't find any nettles). Remove all the liquid by pressing with a clean cloth and fry for five minutes in a little olive oil, then scramble in one or two eggs during the last minute. Season to taste and serve on toast. It's tasty, full of protein, iron and fibre, very filling and totals only 350 calories.

AUTHOR'S NOTE

During my days in the SAS we were sent to the far-flung corners of the world, living for the most part on 'Compo' – tinned rations to the non-military mind. There was no bread with which to eat the canned jam or cheese – so I made my own using an ammunition tin on top of two Primus stoves for an oven. The yeast we had sent in, the flour I begged from the local Arabs, and the rest of the ingredients could be found in the military 'Compo' pack.

MEATS

For years the SAS have maintained a secret love affair with curry. This came about during the long treks into the dark jungles of Borneo where the only food they had was what they carried. For the most part military rations those days consisted primarily of dehydrated and totally tasteless meat. So the odd natural sweet potato, bamboo core, onion or pepper was added along with several spoonful of curry powder. Although military rations have advanced to the point where dehydrated food has been replaced with highly advanced freeze-dried products, the SAS curry culture still remains. As an aid to healthy living, curry can convert vegetables into a tasty and nourishing main meal. This conversion, due to its colour and opacity, helps mask the fact that there is little or no meat in the dish.

Curry is a great way of disguising vegetables to look like meat.

Best Meal: 7 oz (200 g) of lean beef, chicken and/or mixed hard vegetables (potatoes, carrots etc.) cut into cubes.

  1 chopped onion

  1 stock cube

  3 large tablespoons of curry powder

  2½ pints (1.5 litres) of water

Slightly brown the chopped onion in a little olive oil and add the meat and curry powder stirring for about two minutes. Pour into a large saucepan, pour in the water and mix in the stock cube, and bring to the boil. If you wish to add vegetables to bulk it out, add them now and simmer for about two hours, stirring occasionally. Leave overnight so that the curry spices have time to mellow and serve with plain rice. Depending on if you added vegetables or not, this meal will supply four ample servings, which you can either share or freeze for later use. Energy value per serving, including rice, is between 365 and 400 calories.

FITNESS STEW

The one major problem with dieting is the feeling that the food we consume lacks real body – but not with my fitness stew. It looks like a real meal, tastes like a real meal and is highly nutritious. More importantly it will satisfy your hunger and you will have the satisfaction of consuming only fresh ingredients. Try to limit the amount of starchy vegetables you use because the better the mix the better the taste. Prepare as below, its delicious.

Best Meal: one pack of mixed vegetables, or select your own.

> 10½ (300 g) of lean meat, pork, beef or lamb (not chicken)
>
> 2 Oxo cubes.
>
> 2½ pints (1.5 litres) of water.

Chop the vegetables and meat into mouth-sized pieces and add to the water. Crumble the Oxo cubes and bring the whole lot to the boil for five minutes then simmer on a low heat for about two hours. Do not thicken or use extra salt. The meal will provide three large servings, which you can either share or freeze. Energy value per serving is 380 calories.

OUTDOOR EATING

The latter part of this book demands that much of the exercise is conducted outdoors over hilly terrain, where your body will require nourishment to meet the extra energy demand. Eating outdoors is particularly pleasurable especially when you are surrounded by magnificent scenery. Moreover, walking over the hills constitutes arduous exercise with an average calorie burn of between 350 and 450 calories per walking hour, which will increase your daily calorie balance to around 3000. To achieve the best from you outdoor exercise you are advised to eat a normal diet, but one which is also rich in carbohydrates with average protein levels and a low-fat content. This can be achieved by purchasing fresh food and making your own menus. Fresh food for consumption while walking your routes can consist of sandwiches, fruit or a preprepared meat held in a sealed picnic box. If you are still trying to control your weight then fresh food is the way to go.

If you are not trying to control your body weight then you may wish to subscribe to ready-made camping meals. Many people now prefer to carry packs of freeze-dried food (its what the SAS carry) while walking over the hills. This type of food has improved dramatically over the past few years and is ideal for camping due to its light weight. The packs contain 96 per cent real food, as opposed to 80 per cent water in wet foods. They are normally packed in a foil pouch that enables boiling water to be added, thus reconstituting the contents hot in the bag. The food can also be cooked normally on a heat-source and by adding water. Menus include breakfasts, main meals and desserts, and an excellent vegetarian choice is available. Meals take about five minutes to prepare when cooked in the pack and about seven minutes if cooked conventionally. Freeze-dried food has a shelf-life of up to three years.

Always carry a supply of food when walking on mountains. Freeze-dried food is excellent for carrying and cooking while walking over rough terrain.

SUMMARY

Remember regular exercise and a sensible diet is the only way to achieve weight loss. While the initial process may be hard and take quite a long time, the benefits are a healthier and prolonged life. A fitter body also produces a fitter brain, providing clear thought that will help improve your lifestyle. Define your aim, find the determination to achieve it and the confidence to maintain it.

Finally, do not let fitness dominate your life. If there is a special occasion, enjoy yourself, because life without happiness is no life.

CALORIE COUNTER

This table list foods which contain a whole range of nutrients. The figures given are for 3-oz (100-g) portions. The figures have been rounded up or down to the nearest five calories in order to make the calculation of your daily calorie intake easier. Some brand names, presentation and processing methods will alter the product calorie count slightly and it is recommended that you check the item before purchasing.

All Bran	270
Almonds, shelled	550
Apples	50
Avocado	225
Bacon, grilled	405
Banana	79
Beans, baked	75
Beefburger	260
Beef, lean	220
Beef sausages, grilled	260
Beetroot, jar of	30
Biscuits, general	450
Bread, white	230
wholemeal	210
Butter, salted	740
Cake, general	380
Cheese, Cheddar	400
cottage	100
Danish Blue	350
Edam	300
Stilton	450

Chicken, roast skinless	150
roast	220
Chutney	200
Cod in batter	200
steamed/baked	85
Cornflakes	380
Cream, double	450
single	215
Crisps	530
Egg, boiled	150
fried	220
scrambled	230
Ham, cooked sliced	120
Honey, jar of	260
Ice cream	160
Ketchup, tomato	100
Kidneys, fried	150
Lamb chop, grilled	300
Liver, fried	220
Lobster, boiled	120
Margarine, general	700
Flora	540
Marmite/Bovril	200
Milk chocolate	520
Milk, condensed	300
skimmed	33
whole	65
Oil, vegetable	900
Olive oil	900
Onions, pickled	53
Oranges	60
Peaches, canned	85
Peanut butter	620

Peanuts, shelled	400
Peas, frozen	45
tinned	65
Pilchards, tinned	125
Plaice in batter	280
steamed	100
Pork belly, grilled	350
Pork chop, grilled	250
leg roast	286
sausages, grilled	320
Porridge	50
Potato, baked	85
boiled	80
chips	260
Prawns, cooked	110
Rice, boiled	130
Salmon, smoked	140
poached	200
Scampi, fried	320
Spaghetti, boiled	120
Sugar, white	400
Sweetcorn, frozen	120
on the husk	80
Syrup, Golden 1 tin	300
Trout, steamed	130
Tuna, canned	180
Turkey, roast	155
Walnuts, shelled	520
Weetabix	340
Whitebait, fried	500
Yoghurt, fruit	90
low-fat	50

Drinks

Beer, average	30
Cider, sweet	40
Blackcurrant, undiluted	230
Coffee, no milk or sugar	5
Coke	40
Lemonade	25
Liqueurs, average	250
Spirits, average	210
Tea, no milk or sugar	3
Tomato juice	15
Water	0
Wine, average	70

CALORIE USAGE

The calorie count shown below is based on one hour duration of the given sport or activity, this includes inactive time during the anaerobic sports.

Aerobics, traditional	333
Badminton, social	252
Basketball, moderate	392
Bowling, competitive	252
Callisthenics, vigorous	192
Canoeing, 4 mph	276
Chopping wood	252
Cycling, 5 mph	225
10 mph	444

Dance, slow	84
vigorous	252
Gardening	114
Golf	158
Horse riding, trot	195
walk	144
Jogging, 4.5 mph	480
Karate	504
Kitchen work	84
Mountain climbing	420
Racquetball	390
Skipping, 120 rpm	420
Rowing machine	528
Running on the spot	504
Running, 7 mph	588
Skating	192
Skiing, cross-country	504
downhill	420
Soccer	360
Stair climbing	720
Swimming,	
backstroke 20 yds/min	168
breaststroke 20 yds/min	192
crawl 20 yds/min	192
Tennis, social	276
Trampoline	336
Walking	
2 mph	138
3 mph	192
4 mph	246
Waterskiing	480
Weight-training, average	384

COLLINS GEM
BABIES' names

COLLINS GEM
BEER

COLLINS GEM
BIRDS

COLLINS GEM
CALORIE
Counter

COLLINS GEM
FACT FILE

COLLINS GEM
FENG SHUI

COLLINS GEM
FLAGS

COLLINS GEM
Healthy
EATING

COLLINS GEM
QUOTATIONS

COLLINS GEM
SAS
Self-Defence

COLLINS GEM
SAS
Survival Guide

COLLINS GEM
SEASHORE

COLLINS GEM
TREES

COLLINS GEM
Understanding
DREAMS

COLLINS GEM
WILD
flowers

COLLINS GEM
WINE
Dictionary